GOOD BYE BACK PAIN!

GOOD BYE BACK PAIN!

by

Dr. Leonard Faye

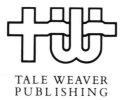

TALE WEAVER
PUBLISHING

LOS ANGELES

Library of Congress Catalog Card Number: 90-71333

ISBN 0-942139 -01

The information in this book is not intended as medical advice. Its intention is solely informational and educational. It is assumed that the reader will consult a medical or health professional should the need for one be warranted.

Tale Weaver Publishing, Los Angeles

ACKNOWLEDGMENTS

Many people have enthusiastically worked together to produce this book. They all knew it would help back pain sufferers become informed health care consumers. I want to give my sincere thanks to Ron Baron and Dick Weaver of Tale Weaver Publishing, Lydia Encinas, associate writer, Michael Faye, photographer, Art Proulx, graphic artist, Neal Hitchens and Charity Staley, models, Gretchen Henkel, editor, and Wong Design, cover layout and design.

TABLE OF CONTENTS

To Bernadette,
my loving wife
and best friend.

Introduction

"Life is Movement . . . Movement is Life."

Your back hurts!

You can't work and you can't relax.

It's hard to sit, it's even worse getting up. Bend? Walk? Run? Pure torture.

But don't worry, you're not alone. Help has arrived.

Each year in the United States, millions of people suffer from a multitude of conditions associated with back ailments. Back pain is as common as the common cold, but with this big difference:

You *can* stop back pain!

It is estimated that back pain-related problems are costing the American public at least $40 billion annually. Even at that enormous cost, it would be money well spent if a cure could be guaranteed. Unfortunately, very few people who suffer from back ailments find any kind of long-lasting relief.

By the time the "classic back pain sufferer" is around 35 years old, he or she has already been to many practitioners with few lasting results. For this person, there was usually a history of a late teens or early twenties incident which caused severe back pain.

If the sufferer sought a doctor's advice, the recommendation was usually to treat the pain with "rest and respect" until it went away. Every year or so it would flare up after some new incident, but each time the discomfort seemed to get worse from doing less. Different doctors would be consulted and all the arthritic diseases would be ruled out.

Because the disease had not progressed to a point requiring surgical intervention, the orthopedist would prescribe physiotherapy and plant the concept to return when surgery was necessary for ultimate relief. His attitude toward physiotherapy would be lukewarm at best and far from encouraging.

After several visits to a physiotherapy department, this classic patient soon found out that he or she could apply heat and do exercises at home. The physiotherapy visits would seem impersonal and such a waste of time.

Inevitably, this poor sufferer had friends who knew of a chiropractor, osteopath, acupuncturist, masseur, hypnotist or herbalist who could cure back pain in one easy visit. The sufferer probably went to anyone who might be able to help, as it became obvious the medical approach was yielding few results. There are more than 85 million back pain sufferers in the United States alone who can attest to that fact!

Because this developing condition is episodic it naturally has its good and bad periods. Almost any treatment during a pain episode will succeed to some extent. However, most treatments will not prevent further episodes. In many cases patients such as our sufferer often get better in spite of the treatments they receive.

Back pain is a symptom. The disease is a process of disc and joint erosion combined with

irregular outgrowths of bone and calcified ligaments. The spinal cord and its branches eventually get involved and become diseased. Back
pain sufferers can experience pain from age 18
to 40 and be unaware of the process in
progress.

The key to long-term results is found in the
treatment given after the pain is cleared. The
abnormal biomechanical function must be elim-
inated and other contributing factors must also
be changed.

Would you sit around with short hamstrings,
weak abdominal muscles, restricted hip joints
and locked spinal joints (to name a few) if you
knew a surgeon was waiting down the line to
offer his services? While these conditions go
untreated, your life is being grossly restricted by
a dull backache that often erupts into a humili-
ating, excruciating, distorting back pain.

If you've been seeing a specialist and have
not yet achieved satisfactory results, or if you
have not yet sought help, then this guide book
is for you. I will explain how you can take
charge of your own back problem, and if necessary, advise you on how to locate the best possible treatment.

Glorious freedom will be awaiting the former
sufferer once he or she knows what the
condition is, and whether the specialist is really
supplying more than temporary relief!

During my 30 years as a back specialist, I
have treated thousands of patients with muscle,
joint and bone problems, but most predominantly, I have treated people suffering from back pain.

My approach is unique and has proved successful in many thousands of individual cases by offering patients (1) education and (2) action. I believe people suffering from back pain can be their own best advisors. That is, the patient should be able to identify the problem, and the patient must be able to select the right professional to get results.

In six simple chapters, this guide book will explain: (1) the causes of back pain, (2) the self-diagnosis of back pain, (3) the professionals who treat back pain, (4) the therapies, (5) home treatment, (6) relaxation techniques.

While other books have been written on this subject, they have most always been written from the specialists' points of view. *Good Bye Back Pain* is written for you — a layperson who wants complete answers in language easy to understand.

The medical community cannot agree on what causes back pain, and certainly not on how to treat this epidemic. I staunchly believe that the millions of sufferers across America and around the world deserve better treatment than being advised to "learn to live with it." I wrote this book to help sufferers realize that what they face is not a hopeless situation.

If you have your health — you have everything. If you are now feeling pain and despair, let me advise you to turn the page and continue reading.

There is a light at the end of the tunnel. It will be my pleasure to guide you there.

●　●　●

Chapter One

The Causes of Back Pain

For every action there is a reaction;
And for every cause there is an effect.

Communicate Your Symptoms

If you currently have back pain, it is vitally important for you to understand the causes clearly, or to be able to describe the various symptoms to your doctor. Poor understanding and vague descriptions will only delay the correct treatment. If you can articulate your symptoms, you can help your doctor help you get better, faster!

Most doctors would agree that a thorough consultation and a carefully recorded case history can almost always guide them to the correct diagnosis. However, some doctors, because of their specialty and training, limit themselves to their particular concept as to the causes of back pain. No matter what you tell them, they are going to prescribe the same treatments they always do.

There are unique causes to all bad backs and no single treatment system succeeds for everyone. The less the doctor or therapist asks you, the more likely you will be slotted into a system. Beware of the doctor who does not listen and ask questions about your back pain: you may become a guinea pig in a treatment mill. Whether it suits you or not is a matter of luck. So make sure you are treated as an individual.

It is amazing that most people lose their memories when they enter the examination room in a doctor's office. They also have a tendency to become monosyllabic and drop all the descriptive words that could better help the doctor comprehend their problem.

Don't take along a written list (the doctor may peg you as a "neurotic"), but make sure you have a list of your symptoms in your mind. Communication from patient to doctor is essential to the diagnostic process. The physical examination and x-rays are only necessary to confirm the diagnosis and to rule out a few rare possibilities.

I can recall treating a non-English speaking patient without an interpreter. He had described where he "used to" get leg pain in minute detail, and I mistakenly thought he was presently suffering from this pain. It turned out after a few weeks he had been describing a pain in his leg he "used to" get all the time, but never experienced after he strained his back. I had missed the "used to" in my translation of his French. Fortunately, once we began communicating on the same level, I was able to solve his problem.

Even if there is no language barrier, don't tell the doctor you have "a hitch in your get along" or a "pain in the back." Describe exactly where things are. Describe the difference between a sharp or dull pain, a constant or intermittent one. Make certain your doctor knows precisely what you are feeling even if he is too busy to investigate it thoroughly. Keep in mind that doctors are human too. It might be difficult for your family doctor to become interested in your back pain when a previous patient was seriously depressed, or had to be told that he or she had a terminal illness.

Remember, a major part of your ability to alleviate back pain is your ability to communicate with your doctor.

How Your Spine Works

To identify the cause of your back problem, it is essential to first understand how the human back works. Once you have a clear picture, you'll be better able to recognize the four major causes of pain. Then managing the problem will be easier.

The spine has three major functions:
1) To support the body,
2) to protect the spinal cord, and
3) to enable the body to move smoothly.

Humans are the only creatures on earth who consistently walk upright upon two legs. Because we are working against gravitational force, there is more stress on our spines, especially in the lower spine area. For this reason, we as a species are more prone to back-related problems.

It is important to understand the mechanics of the back. As an example, imagine that your spine or backbone functions as a bicycle chain. When it's running properly, you can go up hills, across town, or just run along carefree mile after mile. But if you're trying to get around on a chain with several links which are locked or frozen together, you're in a world of hurt.

As with a bicycle chain, if the chain of 24 individual bones and over 75 joints which link your spine together are in any way impaired (not able to move properly), there will be abnormal wear and tear on your back and body. However, unlike a bicycle chain, your spine is composed of many individual components which all must work together in order for your back to function properly.

How Your Spine Is Put Together

The spine is composed of three basic parts:

1) The bony framework consisting of verte- brae and joints,
2) the spinal cord and nerves, and
3) the soft tissues: muscles, ligaments and discs.

The spine has five transitional zones from the head to the tail bone. Two columns run the full length. And although these columns are joined together, they have separate functions. The front part which faces the inside of your body is responsible for support. It consists of block-like structures that are named the Body of the Vertebra.

Single discs lie between each body. Each disc is jelly-like in the center and is surrounded by a wall which keeps it together. The wall is made of webbed fibers that are attached around, above and below the body. Thus, the disc is secured between the two bodies.

The vertebral arch makes up the back part of your spine. It is so named because it forms an arch which houses the spinal cord. The vertebral arch assists in the movement of the back.

To complete this picture of the basic spinal structure, refer to Diagram 1 showing a pair of vertebrae (The Basic Motion Unit) on page 10. Notice how each vertebral arch has two upper and two lower joints. Their surfaces are called facets.

In order to understand how your spine is designed, it may be simpler to just imagine a stack of blocks. Think of the front column made up of blocks with discs in between, and two columns on both sides to the rear composed of slippery joints. We call each of these sets of two blocks a motion unit.

Mother Nature has given us ligaments to keep these neat little stacks from falling apart while moving. Ligaments work much like tiny ropes to guide the movement, while muscles contract to cause the movement.

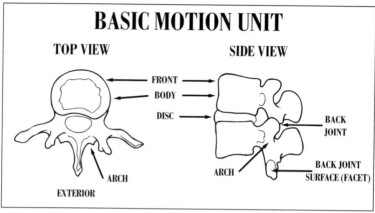

BASIC MOTION UNIT

TOP VIEW   SIDE VIEW

FRONT
BODY
DISC
BACK JOINT
BACK JOINT SURFACE (FACET)
ARCH
EXTERIOR
ARCH

Diagram 1

Finally, our spines curve in a lazy "S" from front to back. This curve is not only normal, it is essential if the spine is to function properly. Of course, too much curve or too little curve will impair movement, too much being more common than too little.

Four Basic Causes of Back Pain

With a basic grasp of how the spine is set up, you will be better able to understand the four basic causes of back pain, which are:

1) MECHANICAL
This category is divided into two groups: dysfunctional, resulting from a repetitive job like a brick-layer's; and traumatic, resulting from an injurious incident such as a car accident.
2) DEGENERATIVE
This refers to pain caused by unhealthy, weak and broken-down tissue which is not able to provide necessary support.

3) SYSTEMIC

This category includes rheumatoid and gouty arthritis, osteoporosis, anemia, allergies, etc., which can cause back pain.

4) STRESS-INDUCED

This can produce muscle spasms that cause restriction of the joints, and a non-stop pain cycle.

Mechanical Back Pain

Chances are that your disorder falls into this category. More than 90% of people suffering back ailments have a mechanical cause of their pain. The main mechanical disorders that lead to back pain are the irregular motion of joints, leg problems, shortened muscles, and of course, physical injury.

MECHANICAL DYSFUNCTION

You have already learned that the basic unit of your back is a motion unit. Most motion units consist of two vertebrae connected by a disc and the two posterior superior and posterior inferior joints.

The disc acts like a rubber ball bearing, allowing the vertebrae to move because the ball can twist and bend along with the vertebral joints. From a mechanical point of view, it is extremely important for the disc to twist and bend without restriction, and for the two joints to be able to slide in the directions necessary for smooth locomotion of the body. If there is any breakdown in the joints' ability to flex forward, extend backward, rotate to the left and right, or to bend sideways to the left and right, then you have the first stage of mechanical dysfunction. In other words, you will experience pain if a joint's ability to move is in any way impaired.

Motion in the lower back is dependent upon flexibility of the pelvic joints. These joints allow the pelvis to transfer mechanical forces from the legs via the hip joint to the lower back spine. If these joints are not able to accommodate flexing, then you will feel stress when performing simple motions. The entire spine and pelvis must be mobile on the hip joints, much like the relationship of the universal joint to the axle of a car, so that the car can move forward or backward. Chapter Two will offer simple tests so you can determine if you have normal hip function or not.

The following is an example of impaired hip functioning. Some years ago, an article appeared in a popular magazine written by a chronic back pain sufferer who had been almost everywhere in an attempt to find relief. The gist of his story was that after many years of suffering with debilitating pain and a limp, he was finally cured when an osteopath pulled his leg and he felt a suction-like "pop" in his hip joint. The back pain cleared because the faulty hip mechanics traumatizing the lower back had been corrected. Many patients have experienced such relief after a hip manipulation or a foot and ankle manipulation.

If your ankle joints are weakened in any way (if they collapse inward rather than stay upright as they should), then the forces of rotation which occur in the leg transfer up to the sacroiliac through the hip and produce a very damaging force in the lumbar spine. The result is pain!

Less common, but related to ankle troubles, are problems with the feet. When the ankle caves in, it can cause fallen arches and other foot disorders.

Muscles not maintained properly through regular use lose their flexibility, and are vulnerable to sudden injury. Muscles can also cause problems when they become shortened due to disuse, misuse, or improper stretching.

How many times have you heard the story about someone who simply bent over to pick up a piece of paper only to injure their back? I hear this story constantly in my practice. It has probably happened to you. I even had one patient who was bending over to sit on the toilet when the pain and spasm struck! These all-too-frequent occurrences happen because we sit too much. Too much sitting causes the large muscles behind the thighs and the small interior muscles in the lower back to shorten. When these muscles are suddenly required to lengthen by the postural change during bending and stooping, they tend to emit a very sharp pain and/or go into spasms. Stretching exercises are vital to avoid this common cause of back pain.

It is significant to note that poor posture is one of the major causes of mechanical back disorders. Postural stress is frequently the result of sitting for a long time in a poor position, or standing or bending incorrectly while working. Several years ago, Lyman Johnston, a Canadian chiropractor, invented the Posture-O-Meter. This device could determine whether a person was standing with the forces of gravity correctly carried by the spine. If the person's weight was too far behind the proper center of gravity, the Posture-O-Meter assigned a number to rate the so-called posterior gravity line. When a group of people were screened, it was shown that over 90% of the back pain sufferers carried their weight too far behind the gravity line. One of our tests in this book (Page 44) actually catches this problem without the use of the Posture-O-Meter.

Sitting improperly is the worst thing you can do to your back, and one of the easiest postures to correct. If you slump in your chair, day after day, the normal hollow that should exist between your back and the chair disappears. The shoulders tend to follow suit and slump forward.

What occurs is a reverse of nature's natural curve in the lower back. Instead of there being a space between your lower back and the chair, the hollow disappears and your lower back touches the chair. In fact, a space appears between your shoulders and the chair. Constant posture reversing puts an incredible stretch on the ligaments and allows the lower back discs to creep backwards and bulge. This creeping action happens quickly and accounts for the back sufferer who suddenly can't rise from an airplane or theater seat. Thus, you not only get a stretched ligament because of the poor posture, you can also get a bulging disc.

When people with this type of posture rise from a sitting position, they compensate by throwing their heads forward, which further increases the reversal of the natural curve. Finally, the day comes when they try to rise and straighten up and they are unable to do so.

INJURY - STRAIN AND SPRAIN

The irregular motion of joints, leg problems and shortened muscles are the main mechanical disorders that lead to back pain. Added to these are the physical forces of injury that result in sprain or strain. These types of traumatic problems can be described as adding injury to mechanical insult.

One thing the medical community agrees on when it comes to back pain is that strains and sprains cause more pain than anything else. Laypersons often confuse these two types of injury. However, there is a big difference between the two.

Strain results when muscles and tendons are stretched beyond their normal capacity. The shooting, severe pain produces more muscle spasm. The spasm also restricts blood circulation, so that the natural toxic by-products of normal muscle activity are not carried away in the bloodstream. This painful cycle can last for days or weeks. In some cases a "trigger point" develops.

A trigger point will assure that the back pain persists and usually causes the development of pain further away from the strained muscle. This new pain can be intensified when the trigger point is stretched or pressed upon. These trigger points can also send numbness and tingling to the distant point in the leg or buttock.

Trigger points are a common complication of strained lower back muscles.

Back *sprain* is different from strain in that it occurs when there is a tearing of the ligaments, tendons or muscle fibers. Lower back muscles do not strain as often as ligaments sprain. During forward bending the back muscles become relaxed and gravity makes you fall into a bent position. At this point you are hanging on your ligaments and vulnerable to sprain, especially if you are twisted to one side and try to lift at the same time.

For this reason, you should bend your knees before you bend over to lift. With bent knees your back remains more upright and allows the muscles to remain contracted, preventing the ligament sprain. If you don't pivot fully on your hip joints, you hang on your ligaments sooner than normal. And if the weight of your upper body, or the weight you are lifting, is too much, a sprain will invariably occur to the lower back joint ligaments.

After a sprain, local swelling occurs over the next 24 hours, causing even more severe pain the following day. Fluid from the injured tissues collects, producing pressure and irritation on nerves, and so another source of pain develops. Then Nature steps in: the muscle fibers around the area contract to form a natural splint around the joint sprain and spasms occur over a wider area as more muscle bundles contract. The bigger the sprain, the greater the muscle spasm.

Sprains can occur from the repetitive stress of poor posture, occupational postures and actions, injury from accidents, unexpected movements such as missing a step, or even sneezing. Sprains are far more serious than strains and normally take more time to heal.

A complication of painful spasms results from sprains or strains of the small but very important *piriformis* muscle. The piriformis muscle is located right where you sit on your buttock. A spasm there can trap the sciatic nerve and cause severe leg pain. If you've injured your piriformis, sitting is painful and you probably keep pushing your thumb into your buttock muscles to ease the spasm. You may feel as if something is wrong with your hip.

One last note on mechanical disorders: if the condition is allowed to persist, your brain may begin to interpret the accompanying restrictions as normal. You could become stuck in your predicament indefinitely. Reversing these conditioned patterns requires specific balance exercises few doctors prescribe.

Degenerative Back Pain

Although this is a separate cause of back pain, in most cases degenerative back pain is actually a progression of the mechanical disorders. It has to do with wear and tear — if something is working incorrectly, then it usually wears out more quickly than if it is working correctly. A simple comparison is the front end of your car. If the wheels are misaligned, then the tires will wear out more quickly, as well as unevenly.

Wear, tear and exercise can frequently be bedfellows. I will never forget the largest calcium bone spurs I ever saw on an x-ray that were jutting out from a pair of lumbar vertebrae. The patient was a physical education instructor who led an aerobics class four times a day almost every day of the week. His back pain only came on when he had a few days off. This pattern lasted for years. When he worked at exercising and stretching he got relief from the pain. During vacations he suffered with a bad back.

The explanation of his problem involves a paradox. It has been shown that exercising with faulty mechanics establishes a natural compensating muscle splint. This natural splint needs a daily workout to maintain its supporting action. In the meantime, because the mechanics are faulty, the production of a more permanent splint in the form of calcium spurs is stimulated. The wear and tear and inflammation eventually lead to the buildup of calcium deposits, which then develop into little spurs that jut out from the edges of the joints. The boney outgrowth and calcification of ligaments create large permanent spurs.

The moral of this story is to make sure you are exercising with normal mechanical movement. All the joints in your pelvis and spine must be mobile with no lock-ups. Exercise can be a double-edged sword, and using exercise for pain relief will only lead to severe degenerative changes before you know it. Joints which aren't functioning in a mechanically correct manner will wear out the cartilage, and the ligaments and surrounding tissues will become absorbed in the destructive process. This deterioration is sometimes accompanied by painful inflammation. It's like hitting your thumb with a hammer. It becomes painful to touch after the trauma, whereas normally you could squeeze your thumb without pain. The changing inflamed areas of your back can't take the pressure of compression.

The whole degenerative process is full of such painful scenarios, and in most cases, much unnecessary suffering.

Systemic Back Pain

This category refers to disorders which affect the back and other parts of the body simultaneously.

ARTHRITIC CONDITIONS

Foremost on the list of systemic disorders is *rheumatoid arthritis.*

Let's look at these terms separately. Rheumatic diseases affect the connective tissues of the body, often striking the spine. Arthritis (from *arthr* = joint and *itis* = inflammation) literally means the inflammation of a joint.

Inside the affected joints, the cartilage thins out and space narrows with deterioration as the disease progresses. This degeneration causes the release of chemicals which prolong and advance the condition.

Rheumatoid arthritis is considered an autoimmune disease. That is, the system's antibodies, which normally protect against disease, go berserk and gradually begin eating away at the diseased joints. Stress and other emotional factors play a large part in generating this condition.

Blood tests can monitor the rheumatoid activity and rheumatologists have many treatment plans to suit individual sufferers. Some researchers feel diet plays an important part in this systemic disease. Drugs can often control and contain the damage to joints and in many instances, the condition will stop with time.

If your chronic back pain is of a dull, nagging, constant nature, you may have arthritic symptoms. If you've had treatment for the pain without adequate response but the pain does respond to aspirin, then you may have reason to suspect that you have one of the varieties of arthritic conditions.

Interestingly, systemic disorders are not limited to older people. For men, *ankylosing spondylitis*, a form of rheumatoid arthritis, can begin in the early 20s. The first sign of this condition is a dull back pain which gets worse with activity and becomes increasingly sharper. Later, it is accompanied by severe fatigue, irritability and increased pain after any aggressive physical or manipulative therapy.

The disease causes widespread inflammation of the spinal joints, and starts in the sacroiliac pelvic joints. No one is sure of the cause of ankylosing spondylitis, but it is characterized by the following: a flattening of the hollow of the lower back, a loss of forward and backward bending, stiffness of the spinal joints, and a constant, nagging, aching pain that only an anti-inflammatory drug can relieve.

The progression of this disease often occurs because ankylosing spondylitis is one of the most misdiagnosed of back conditions. Left unchecked, it will cause the back to stiffen and the vertebrae to fuse together.

Young men can suffer with this pain into their late 20s and early 30s before its cause is properly diagnosed. Fortunately, ankylosing spondylitis can be slowed considerably with anti-inflammatory drugs and treatment, including daily exercise sessions on a stationary bicycle.

CONTRIBUTING FACTORS

Despite today's great technical advances in the healing arts, the incidence of arthritis in all its varied forms, along with many other degenerative diseases, is not decreasing. Over the years there have been many studies showing that a less stressful environment, more physical exertion and natural foods can produce a population with less degenerative disease. Many factors contribute to the development of degenerative diseases; attending to as many as possible makes good sense. It always seemed odd to me that a person would take an anti-inflammatory drug for an inflamed joint and not address the contributory causes of the inflammation. Psychiatrists and clinical psychologists are rarely recommended for chronic degenerative back pain, yet they can be a big help in a number of stress-related cases. I've had the cooperation of many patients who have improved their eating and living patterns and thus stopped a degenerative disease.

Smoking cigarettes interferes with the absorption of important C vitamins, and taking birth control pills interferes with vitamin B absorption; both B and C are necessary to heal inflammation. I can assure you that the average American diet is not healthy, and our backs suffer from the inadequate intake of vitamins, minerals and protein. Most people eat far too many saturated animal fats that are also linked to heart disease and cancer.

Healthy joints and discs need quality protein. Make sure you eat some real, good old-fashioned, unrefined, unadulterated, natural, raw or lightly cooked food every day. Eat less, and make sure what you eat is high quality. You really are what you eat.

Anemia is another cause of systemic back pain. This pain is also accompanied by the classic signs of fatigue, loss of energy and irritability. If caught in time, anemia can be treated.

OSTEOPOROSIS/PREGNANCY

More than 25% of all post-menopausal women suffer from *osteoporosis*. This condition causes the bones of the spine to become very brittle and vulnerable to compression and fracture. The causes of osteoporosis in older women are still not fully understood, but the disease affects the entire body, especially the backbone.

One widely held theory postulates that the absence of the hormone estrogen is the cause.

Women who suffer from osteoporosis will often improve bone density when taking estrogen and a combination of vitamins and minerals. Increasing your weight-bearing exercise is also essential, as taking estrogen or calcium without exercising is much less effective.

One cause of systemic back pain requiring a special approach is pregnancy. More than 50% of pregnant women will get back pain from their fifth month of pregnancy on. Twenty-five percent of these women suffer daily, though most suffer on a weekly basis. And 65% of these mothers-to-be have severe back pain during labor.

Back pain is most likely if a pregnant woman has developed spinal mechanical dysfunctions before she is pregnant. The increased abdominal weight up front, and the presence of a hormone called *relaxin* (which produces relaxation of the pubis), combine to create many problems. For example, if one sacroiliac joint of the pelvis freezes up, the other pelvic joints will become over-stretched and inflamed as they try to compensate.

The catch-22 is that the unborn baby can be adversely affected if the pregnant woman takes drugs to relieve her pain. However, a study in Sweden showed that seven out of ten prenatal back pain sufferers received complete relief from manipulation alone, without using drugs.

After the birthing process, the hormone relaxin gradually leaves the system and the pelvic and lower back ligaments lose their extra elasticity and tighten up. If the joints are not functioning properly as they tighten, postnatal back pain occurs.

Manipulation is often necessary during and after pregnancy. All women preparing to give birth should be checked by a chiropractor or osteopath for proper biomechanics of the pelvis and lower back. Normal, fully mobile sacroiliac joints make for easier engaging of the baby's head into the birthing canal during delivery.

Examining for pelvic mobility is simple and should be included in the obstetrician's prenatal procedure, although often it is not. It's ironic because during the 1940s and 1950s obstetricians did more sacroiliac research than did orthopedists. The orthopedists believed the sacroiliac joints did not move. But chiropractors, osteopaths and obstetricians knew they did, and they knew they moved quite freely.

Any woman suffering from postpartum back or groin pain should see a chiropractor or an osteopath, either of whom will examine for *symphysis pubis joint instability* which often occurs after birthing. This pelvic joint instability causes very harsh sacroiliac pain along with tenderness of the normally stable pubic joint.

A healthy person does not suffer from systemic disease. All systemic back disorders, including gout and psoriasis, are usually accompanied by changes in one's general health. Many cancers rear their ugly heads initially as back pain. These are characterized by tenderness and local pain which is constant and unaffected by rest or activity, and usually accompanied by fatigue and loss of appetite. These cancers of the spine can be detected by bone-scan, x-ray, or blood tests, and if caught in time can often be treated effectively.

Incidents of back pain caused by *Lyme disease* are on the rise. Lyme disease is a disorder contracted from being bitten by a deer tick which carries the disease bacteria. It's not as unusual as it sounds because of the many wilderness and camping areas in America with deer populations. People visiting or living in these areas (especially the northeastern U.S.) run the risk of being bitten and infected.

There are many other less common systemic diseases. If your back pain is accompanied by a decline in your overall health, you should consult your doctor as soon as possible. Systemic diseases should not be treated at home without a doctor's supervision.

Stress-Induced Back Pain

Most specialists will agree that stress is a major contributor to many back disorders. Stress causes a hormonal change in the body's makeup. Worry, fear, hate, anger, frustration and pent-up emotions cause chemical reactions in the brain, triggering a chain of events that can result in muscle spasm and pain. The acute, severe pain of muscle spasm leads to more anxiety and stress, which in turn cause more muscle spasms, and more pain. It's all a vicious cycle.

I once treated and counseled a man who had never had a back pain in his life — until he arranged to see his 21-year-old daughter for the first time in 19 years. The day after he bought his airplane tickets, he began experiencing a terrible shooting pain which doubled him over and almost immobilized him. Of course he missed his flight, but he did recover in a few weeks.

Then, three weeks later, on the day before he was to fly out again, he had his second disabling back attack.

DISTRESS CYCLE

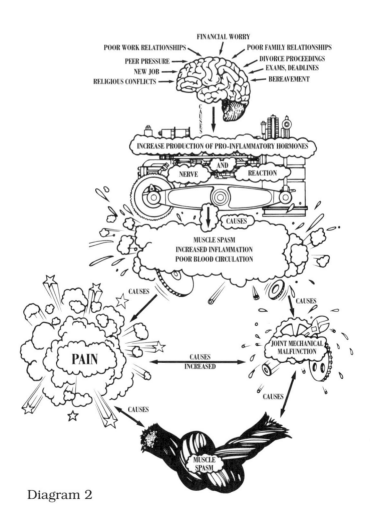

Diagram 2

Apparently the man's guilt and fear about seeing his daughter caused a spill-over of tension into his lower back muscles. In Latin, *soma* refers to muscle. Some emotions are suppressed and express themselves in the soma and hence the term "psychosomatic back pain."

On many occasions, I have treated patients who experienced immediate reversal of the locked joint and muscle spasm. Upon feeling this painless release, the patient oftentimes will begin crying emotionally and uncontrollably for several minutes. And just as often, the patient will have no idea as to the origin of these feelings.

If you have experienced these effects after a chiropractic, osteopathic or physiotherapy treatment, you should also seek counseling. Don't let the suppressed emotions become ulcers, colitis, a ruptured disc, or even a heart attack. Stress can increase the effects of pre-existing systemic, mechanical or degenerative causes of back pain.

It's not difficult to recognize stress-related mechanical dysfunction. Stress sufferers frequently perspire. They have cold hands and feet, are easily startled, fatigued but not sound sleepers, have indigestion and are often acutely aware of their hearts beating. They are edgy and have poor concentration. They react to situations rather than respond thoughtfully. In other words, they are completely distressed.

See the diagram on the opposite page which shows the cycle of stress, muscle spasm, joint dysfunction and mechanical disorders.

In these pages you have seen many causes of back pain. In the next chapter you will identify which is the most likely cause of your own back pain. In our next chapter you also will be able to determine, through a simple test of a few questions, if you're one of the fortunate many who may be able to treat your own back pain, after very little help from the correct professional.

• • •

Chapter Two

Self-Diagnosis

"To be forewarned can set you free."

Faulty biomechanics and poor posture are the most common causes of back pain, and are the easiest to correct. This chapter will show you the difference between good and bad posture and normal versus abnormal mechanics.

The illustrations and tests included here will give you the opportunity to analyze yourself. You will be able to determine what type of back pain you have and evaluate your posture rating.

Taking the necessary steps to correct bad posture habits can alleviate some back pain. It can also save you the disappointment and financial losses of failed treatments.

Chances are you're sitting incorrectly at this very moment. Chances are, also, that your poor posture is a contributing factor to your back pain. The fact is, most people fall into a pattern of improperly sitting, standing and lying without even realizing that these activities are stressing the back joints and shifting the weight and force of gravity away from the discs, where it belongs.

It is easy to fall into poor posture habits. Fortunately, by learning and using corrected biomechanics, it is quite possible to change these bad habits. The first step is the hardest. You have to become aware that these habits exist. To do that, you're going to have to be completely honest with yourself.

Do not downplay your symptoms. A tough, hardy pig farmer once told me his back pain had started six months previously when he had bent over in a field. He had felt a sharp, sudden pain right in the middle of one cheek of his buttocks. The pain made him limp around for a few days, then it lessened to a constant dull ache. After six months he realized the pain wasn't going to go away, so he came to see if I could help him. To the amazement of both of us, an x-ray revealed the head of a bullet was suspended in his buttock muscles. That farmer was the ultimate sufferer.

After answering the following self-assessment questionnaire, you will discover your back pain has many causes. Some you can treat with self-help methods, while others will require that you see the appropriate back specialist for treatment.

Self-Assessment Quiz

This is one test you don't have to study for. So relax (hopefully while sitting in the right position!) and get ready to categorize your own particular back pain. Some of the questions require you to refer to specific photos or diagrams to try out positions. Other questions require that you satisfy both, or all, conditions of the question in order to answer YES.

1. Are you over 40 years of age and experiencing your first constant back pain which came on for no apparent reason?

☐ YES or ☐ NO

2. Do you have constant back pain that is only relieved by the use of aspirin or other arthritis painkillers?

☐ YES or ☐ NO

3. Is your constant back pain or ache accompanied by the need to urinate much more frequently than usual?

☐ YES or ☐ NO

4. Is your back pain or ache accompanied by great fatigue, loss of appetite and/or weight loss?

☐ YES or ☐ NO

5. Ever since a certain incident, has your back pain radiated to your genitals and did they also become numb?

☐ YES or ☐ NO

6. Ever since a certain incident, has your back pain become much more severe and does it radiate down your leg to your foot, accompanied

by occasional or constant numbness?

☐ YES or ☐ NO

7. Ever since a certain incident, has your back pain become worse and have you developed difficulty in urinating or becoming sexually aroused?

☐ YES or ☐ NO

8. Do you have leg pain and notice that your foot catches on the ground quite often?

☐ YES or ☐ NO

9. If you have pain in one leg, try sitting down and raising the good leg straight out, parallel to the floor, as shown in Figures 1 and 2. Do you feel pain in either your lower back or your bad leg?

☐ YES or ☐ NO

10. Is your back pain accompanied by swelling in the back or legs?

☐ YES or ☐ NO

11. Has your back pain constantly persisted for more than one year?

☐ YES or ☐ NO

12. Do you have pains in both legs at the same time?

☐ YES or ☐ NO

13. Do you have numbness in either of your thighs?

☐ YES or ☐ NO

14. Does pain in your leg or back start after you walk a certain distance and is it relieved by resting a short time?

☐ YES or ☐ NO

15. Do you have great difficulty when trying to walk on your toes or heels?

☐ YES or ☐ NO

continued on page 34

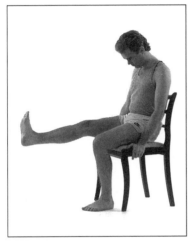 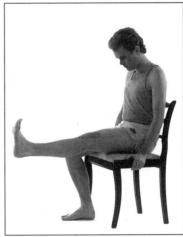

Fig. 1   Fig. 2

This is a test for lumbar disc herniation. The right or left painful leg is resting, the knee bent with the foot flat on the floor. The pain-free leg is straightened. If attempting this maneuver causes back pain that increases when you nod your head forward, you need to see a doctor.

16. Do you have severe leg pain without back pain?

☐ YES or ☐ NO

If you answered YES to one or more of the questions in this first group, it is important that you seek a doctor's opinion as soon as possible. You have a serious complication to one of the four groups of back pain (mechanical, degenerative, systemic, stress-induced). You'll need a prime-contact doctor; an osteopathic, chiropractic or medical doctor is best at this point. If you already have a family doctor or internist, that is the best place to start.

If your answers were NO to all of the previous questions, then your next step is to take the following tests in order to determine your specific type of back pain. Once you know what you have, and what the contributing causes are, then you can sensibly select the correct home care and professional advisor to stop that back pain for good!

If you did answer NO to all the questions above, you are among the 90% of back pain sufferers who have mechanical disorders which cause reactive inflammation, muscle spasm and pain. These conditions are divided into the following groups:

1. Disc related
2. Back joint related
3. Sacroiliac joint related
4. Muscular

Sometimes a sufferer has more than one area of inflammation and therefore is suffering from more than one condition at the same time. All these conditions improve quickly if caught early and can even be effectively treated if they are chronic. In order to determine which group you are in, it is necessary for you to answer the following questions. You could score less than the full number of points required for each diagnosis. However, most likely you will score high in one area. If you score high in more than one area, then you have more than one problem. This is not uncommon.

Test for Mechanical Group One: Disc Syndrome (Non-herniated)

1. Does your back pain increase if you cough, sneeze or bend forward, or if you just bend your head forward, chin to chest?

☐ YES or ☐ NO

2. Does sleeping relieve your back and/or leg pain, and after being up for a few minutes, does the pain return?

☐ YES or ☐ NO

3. Does sitting increase back and/or leg pain?

☐ YES or ☐ NO

4. When lying on your back on the floor, are you unable to raise your painful leg more than 15" off the ground? (See Figures 3, 4, and 5.)

☐ YES or ☐ NO

5. Lie face down with your shoulders raised and supported by a pillow for 15 minutes, as shown in Figure 6. Does the leg pain stop and the pain center in the lower back?

☐ YES or ☐ NO

6. When standing, are you forced to hunch forward and/or to one side?

☐ YES or ☐ NO

7. Does your back pain radiate into your buttock on one side and go down the outside back of your thigh?

☐ YES or ☐ NO

8. Is the range of motion in your lower back greatly restricted or does your back lock up at certain points?

☐ YES or ☐ NO

Scoring

Score 2 points for each YES answer to the previous questions. If you scored 10 or more, you most likely have a disc syndrome.

Test for Mechanical Group Two: Back Joint Syndrome

1. Is the pain in your back in a specific area and to one side?

☐ YES or ☐ NO

2. Does your pain radiate to the back of the thigh of one leg?

☐ YES or ☐ NO

continued on page 38

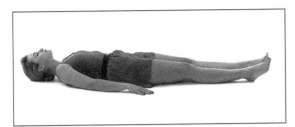

Fig. 3

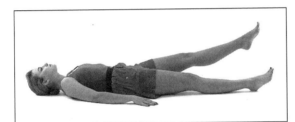

Fig. 4

When a disc has pro- truded, but not necessar- ily herniated or ruptured, neither the sufferer nor a friend can raise the painful leg past 20 degrees (about 15 inches) from the floor.

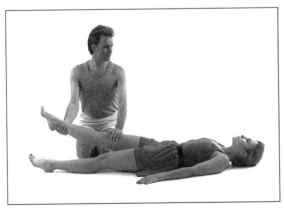

Fig. 5

3. Can you ease the pain by bending slightly forward?

☐ YES or ☐ NO

4. Does the pain intensify if you bend backwards?

☐ YES or ☐ NO

5. Lie on your back as shown in Figures 7 and 8. Can you or a friend raise your leg off the floor to 75 degrees or more before you feel any back pain?

☐ YES or ☐ NO

Scoring

☐   Score 2 points for each YES answer to the previous group of questions. If you scored eight or more, you most likely have an inflamed back joint.

Test for Mechanical Group Three: Sacroiliac Syndrome

1. Is the pain very low on one side of the lower back and does it radiate to the front, side and back of the thigh?

☐ YES or ☐ NO

2. Does your range of motion feel more restricted in the hip joint than in the back?

☐ YES or ☐ NO

3. While lying on your back as shown in Figures 9 and 10, do you feel pain when you or a friend raise your legs between 30 to 60 degrees off the floor?

☐ YES or ☐ NO

continued on page 40

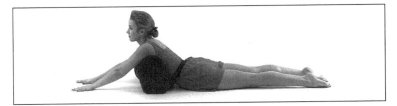

Fig. 6

A *New Zealand physiotherapist discovered this test by accidentally leaving a back and leg pain sufferer in this posture for 15 minutes or so. The leg pain disappeared and centered more in the lower back. If you have leg pain, try it. If your leg pain moves towards your back and is less far down your leg after 15 minutes, rejoice! You should get better and stay better, with the suggestions in this book.*

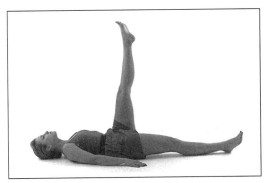

Fig. 7

When you or a friend raise your leg to this height, the pelvis tips and flattens the hollow in your lower back. As this lower back movement occurs, the inflamed back joint starts to feel painful. If raising the leg causes leg pain or a tight pull at the back of your leg, this test has uncovered other problems which will be discussed later.

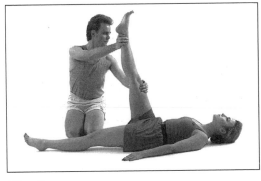

Fig. 8

4. Lying on your back as in Figure 11, bend your painful leg at the knee with the outside of the ankle crossed over the other straightened leg. Do you feel pain in the lower back when you push your bent leg towards the floor?

☐ YES or ☐ NO

5. Upon awakening, is your back very stiff, causing you to get out of bed with difficulty, and then does your back loosen up and get better as the day goes on?

☐ YES or ☐ NO

Scoring

Score 2 points for each YES answer to the previous group of questions. If you scored eight or more, you most likely have a sacroiliac joint problem.

Test for Mechanical Group Four: Muscle Syndrome

1. Does putting pressure on the deeper layer of muscles in the lower back refer the pain to the groin, back and front of the thigh?

☐ YES or ☐ NO

2. When lying down, can you or a friend raise your legs one at a time to 90 degrees with no back pain?

☐ YES or ☐ NO

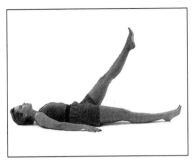
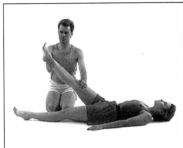

Fig. 9   Fig. 10

Raising your leg or having your leg raised to 60 degrees will cause sacroiliac joint pain. The back pain will occur before the lumbar spine flattens to the floor. The pain will be very low and to the side, almost to the hip joint.

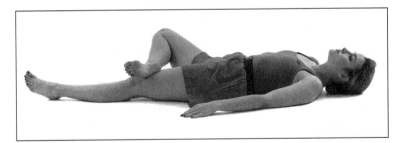

Fig. 11

Place the leg that's on the same side as your lower back pain across your straightened leg and form a figure four (4). If pressing your bent knee to the floor increases your lower back pain, it is most likely your sacroiliac joint is inflamed. If you can't do this test because your bent knee is stuck up in the air, you have a hip joint problem that is probably playing havoc with your lower back pain condition.

3. By probing with care, can you locate the muscle that hurts, and by pressing on a certain spot in the muscle for a few minutes, find relief?

□ YES or □ NO

Scoring

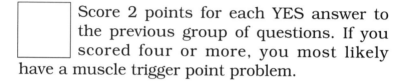

Score 2 points for each YES answer to the previous group of questions. If you scored four or more, you most likely have a muscle trigger point problem.

You may have discovered through the above scoring that your back pain originates from more than one of the above conditions. This is not uncommon. Each condition will need to be treated specifically by your health practitioner. However, the home care exercises and stretches presented in this book will help alleviate all conditions.

If you are one of the majority of back pain sufferers in the mechanical category, the next chapter will help you choose the correct practitioner, or be assured that your present practitioner is right for your type of pain. Then again, you may discover that home care is all you need and use the treatments in Chapter Four.

However, before we move on you also need to assess your posture and muscle/joint flexibility. Lack of good posture and/or poor muscle/joint flexibility will adversely affect your ability to achieve lasting results in the treatment of your back pain. Once again, you must answer YES or

NO. A NO reply here will mean poor posture or loss of flexibility is involved in your back problem, even if a lifting incident initiated the first pain.

Posture, Muscle/Joint Tests

1. When looking at yourself in a full-length mirror, do your shoulders and hips appear to be level?

☐ YES or ☐ NO

2. While standing in a relaxed manner, as shown in Figures 12 and 13, can you raise up onto your toes without rocking forward? (Figure 13 is normal.)

☐ YES or ☐ NO

3. Refer to Figures 14, 15 and 16. Can you sit on your heels (squat) with your feet parallel and a foot apart while leaving your heels on the ground? (Figures 14 and 15 are normal; Figure 16 is incorrect.)

☐ YES or ☐ NO

4. While standing with your feet slightly apart and parallel, can you lean forward with straight legs and touch your toes?

☐ YES or ☐ NO

5. While standing (feet slightly apart and parallel), can you lean backward without twisting and touch the back of each knee?

☐ YES or ☐ NO

6. While standing (feet slightly apart and parallel), can you lean to each side without twisting and reach to the outside of each knee?

☐ YES or ☐ NO

continued on page 46

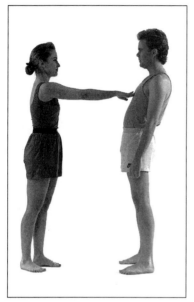

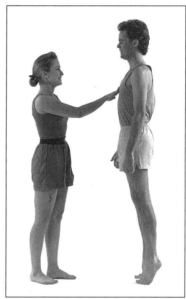

Fig. 12   Fig. 13

Ninety percent of back pain sufferers stand with too much weight on their back joints instead of forward onto the discs where it belongs. To see if this is one of your problems, have someone lightly place a finger on your chest bone. If you have to rock forward a few inches before you can raise up onto your toes (Figure 12), you have this bad posture problem. Good posture is standing at that point where you can rise up onto your toes without rocking forward, as in Figure 13.

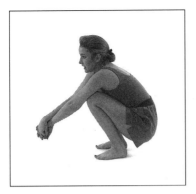

Fig. 14

In countries where people squat as in Figures 14 and 15, there is much less degenerative disc disease at the age of 55. If your flexibility is not good enough you will squat incorrectly, as in Figure 16. Learn to squat correctly by holding onto a counter top or sink front, making sure your heels stay flat on the floor. This stretch is a real winner. Persist until you can comfortably squat this way for a few minutes.

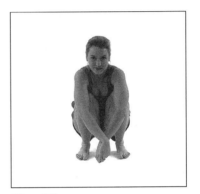

Fig. 15

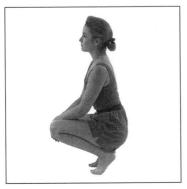

Fig. 16

7. When lying on your back with your hip flexed 90 degrees and your lower leg parallel to the floor, can you then straighten your lower leg so the entire leg is perpendicular to the floor? See Figures 17, 18, and 19. (Figure 18 shows how the leg should straighten.)

☐ YES or ☐ NO

8. While lying on your back, can you pull your knee to your chest while your straight leg remains flat on the floor? Refer to Figures 20 and 21 for illustration. (Figure 20 shows that the leg should not bend at the knee.)

☐ YES or ☐ NO

9. When lying face down, can you bend your knee, and pull it in so that your heel hits your buttock? (Figures 22, 23, and 24.)

☐ YES or ☐ NO

10. Lying face down as shown in Figure 25, can you lift your arms and legs off the floor at the same time?

☐ YES or ☐ NO

11. Lying face up, can you do a knees-bent sit-up without anchoring your feet? (Figure 26).

☐ YES or ☐ NO

12. Lying on your side with your feet anchored, can you raise your shoulders 10 to 12 inches off the floor? Figure 27 correctly demonstrates this diagnostic exercise.

☐ YES or ☐ NO

13. Sit on the floor with the bottoms of your feet together as shown in Figure 28. Can you easily bring your knees close to the floor?

☐ YES or ☐ NO

continued on page 53

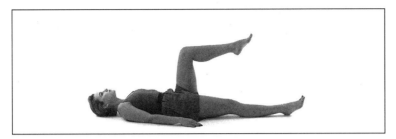

Fig. 17

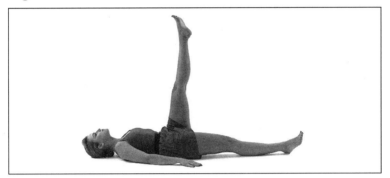

Fig. 18

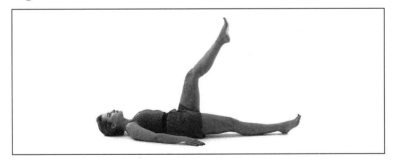

Fig. 19

The hamstring muscles at the back of your thigh should be long enough to allow you to straighten your leg from the position in Figure 17 to the position in Figure 18. If your leg does not straighten, guesstimate the number of degrees short of straightening. The bigger the angle away from a straight leg, the shorter your hamstrings. The shorter your hamstrings, the more likely it is that they are affecting your back pain. It is tantamount to malpractice to be treated for a bad back and not be getting help for short hamstrings!

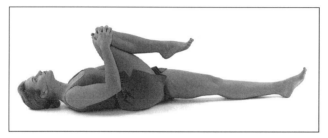

Fig. 20

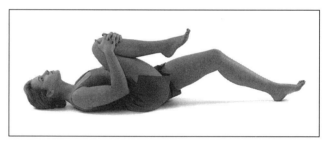

Fig. 21

The large and very powerful hip flexor muscle (psoas muscle, pronounced SO-AS) anchors to your lower back vertebrae and becomes a major factor in faulty lower back mechanics. If the psoas muscle is too short, you cannot keep the opposite leg relaxed and extended flat on the floor, while you pull one knee towards your chest.

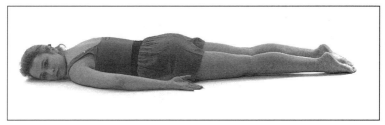

Fig. 22

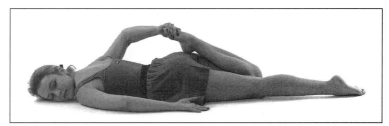

Fig. 23

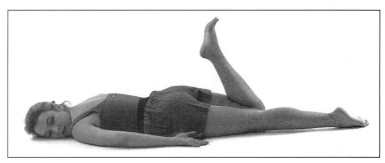

Fig. 24

The large quadricep muscles (called "quads") that form the front of your thigh should be long enough to allow you to easily place your heel on your buttock while lying face down. The shorter your quads, the further your heel will be from your buttock and the more likely it will be that this is a part of your lower back problem.

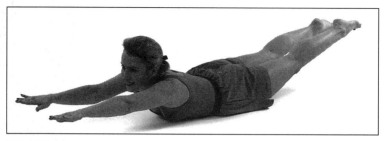

Fig. 25

In chronic lower back pain sufferers, the extension muscles are weak. You should be able to easily hold your hands and feet in the air at the same time for a count of 10. You will need electric muscle stimulation to tone these muscles if your back is painful and inflamed. If this exercise does not produce a lingering pain, you can commence our recommended extension exercises.

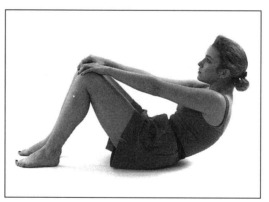

Fig. 26

Because your back is hurting, test the strength of your abdominal muscles with a gentle sit-up. Hold the above sit-up for 10 seconds and then let yourself down to the floor slowly. If you can't hold your rib cage off the floor without using your arms or anchoring your feet, you need to considerably strengthen your abdominal muscles.

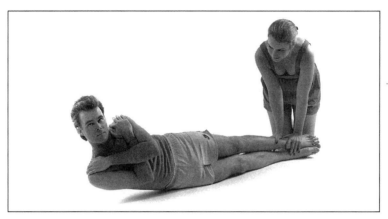

Fig. 27

The most important muscle stabilizer for the lower back is the lateral bending muscle called the quadratus lumborum, or QL muscle. Chronic back pain sufferers rarely have strong QL muscles. Before you try to lift yourself up side-ways, make sure your upper shoulder does not rotate backwards. This cheating action will use the abdominals. Some famous athletes I have treated for chronic back pain could not do this exercise. You should be able to lift your bottom shoulder 10-12 inches off the floor.

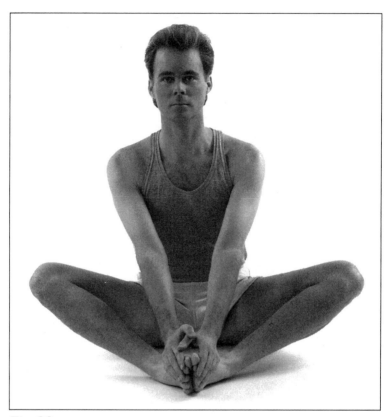

Fig. 28

This posture determines if your hip joints are flexible enough to have a pain-free back. If you cannot bring one or both knees close to the floor, either the groin muscles are too short or your hip joint is restricted. A doctor will need to determine whether one or both is the case. The good news is that you can change the range of motion in both cases. The bad news is that it takes perseverance over many months, often with professional help. Difficulty with this position reveals a significant finding. Don't ignore it.

14. Stand straight and at ease. Look down at your ankles. Are the two bands of Achilles tendons perpendicular to the floor?

☐ YES or ☐ NO

15. Take a look at your kneecaps. Are they pointing forward like the headlights of a car?

☐ YES or ☐ NO

Scoring

A NO answer to *any* of the previous group of questions indicates you have a posture problem or shortened and/or weakened muscles. Not correcting these faults is foolish. These are the problems that cause the recurrence of back pain. Chapter Five describes how you can work to correct them.

Pain may be the reason you cannot easily perform some of these actions. If you are presently under professional care, and you are not working at correcting these shortened muscles and restricted joints, it is highly unlikely you will be able to stop your back pain for very long. You probably will continue to experience episodes of acute pain or attacks until a surgical crisis occurs or old age solves the problem with a natural fusion of the bones.

Look at the charts on the next page. These will enable you to see how you compare to desirable postures. Having a friend help you would be useful, but a full-length mirror will also do.

Turn sideways. Stand in your usual posture. If your belly is flat, you're in good shape. If your stomach protrudes but your back is nearly straight, you're still in fine shape. However, if you have a "pot belly" and an exaggerated hollow in the lower area of your back, then you're in trouble.

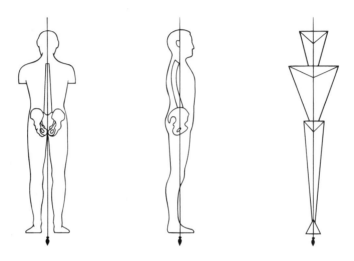

Vertical line represents gravity in normal standing posture.

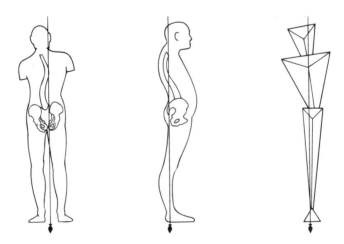

In abnormal posture, vertical line moves off center.

Now look at your head. If it's being carried high above the shoulders, that's great. Your head should not be hanging low out in front of your shoulders. Poor head/neck posture causes stress in the lower back region, further complicating the recovery cycle.

At this juncture you should be able to identify the cause of your back pain problem. If you're still not sure, go back and review the first two chapters. Take the next step in selecting the correct professional only after you are certain of the cause of your ailment.

Diagnosis Summary

Non-Mechanical and Severe Disc Syndrome:

If you answered YES to one or more questions from the first group of questions on pages 31-34, you must go to a chiropractor, medical or osteopathic doctor.

Mechanical Conditions and Their Symptoms

1. DISC SYNDROME:
Back and leg pains get worse as the day progresses. Your back locks up at certain points. Flexing your neck forward hurts your lower back. You can't raise your legs off the ground while they are straight.

2. BACK JOINT SYNDROME:

The back pain is over a specific spot and to one side. The pain eases when you bend slightly forward. Bending backward to one side increases the pain, which also may radiate to the back of one thigh.

3. SACROILIAC SYNDROME:

The pain is very low to one side of the lower back and radiates to the front, side and back of the thigh. You wake up almost unable to get out of bed. Then, as the day goes on, and you walk around, the pain eases.

4. MUSCLE SYNDROME:

You can dig around with your thumb and find the exact spot that causes your pain, and it radiates when you press on it. Continued deep pressure gives relief in a minute.

• • •

Chapter Three:

The Professionals

"Admire the person who seeks the truth.
Beware the person who has found it."

Finding the right professional or specialist to treat your particular back pain is the single most important thing you can do in order to successfully overcome your problem. This chapter explains what the many different specialists offer. By understanding the orientation of each specialist, you will be able to find the proper practitioner to help you with your particular ailment. Although you will follow the guidelines of your primary care practitioner, it will be up to you to have control over your own treatment plan.

Family Practitioner / Internist

Most people with minor back problems first seek the help of the family doctor. Whether they receive the correct care is highly speculative. A family practitioner or internist may be able to provide adequate treatment in many cases. However, a responsible doctor should be able to recognize a back ailment immediately, and know whether he or she can treat it, or whether the patient should be referred to a proper specialist.

Most family practitioners are able professionals, but they are not specialists. You wouldn't think of going to your family doctor for a prescription for new glasses. Of course, you'd seek the advice of an ophthalmologist or optometrist. The same thing applies to those suffering from back problems. If it is nothing more than a simple strain, then the family doctor may indeed be able to provide adequate help. However, with cases involving less obvious causes, there are limitations where family practitioners or even internists are concerned.

A good family practitioner should know his or her limitations. After having tried but failed to successfully treat persistent back pain, he or she should advise you to seek another professional. Normally, pills only mask the effects of persistent back pain, and do not treat the underlying causes. Prescribing medication without treating the cause of the pain is tantamount to turning off the fire alarm and then leaving the scene of the fire.

• • •

The following questions/comments should be discussed and/or answered by your family practitioner who is looking after your back pain:

1. Have enough tests been ordered to determine whether the back pain is systemic or mechanical?

2. What is the diagnosis? (Check this against the questionnaire in the previous chapter.)

3. Is the cause being treated, or are you receiving painkillers to suppress the symptoms?

4. If you are not getting the cause treated, ask for a referral to a recommended specialist. The specialist should deal with correcting the causes. (See further ahead in this chapter for comments on chiropractors, orthopedists, osteopaths and physiotherapists, etc.)

5. Does your family doctor immediately refer you to an orthopedist? If you know you have mechanical back pain which is not an operative disc problem, do not waste your time and money seeing an orthopedist. Manipulation of the locked joints, anti-inflammatory treatment of the inflamed tissues and stretching of the shortened muscles and ligaments is the regimen of choice. These conservative measures are the norm for many modern doctors of chiropractic, osteopaths, specially-trained physiotherapists and the rare medical manipulator.

6. Does your family practitioner or internist object to the idea of manipulation? If he or she is unaware of recent research studies conducted in the U.S., Canada, England and a few non-English speaking countries, which show the

value of manipulation, it is time to take matters into your own hands and change doctors.

Orthopedist / Orthopedic Surgeon

The role of the orthopedist is to determine whether or not the patient is a candidate for surgery, or whether he or she should be referred to a physical therapist.

It is a well-known fact that back surgery leads the list of unnecessary surgical procedures. Recent Canadian research indicates that only two to three percent of chronic back pain sufferers actually need surgery! The other 97% to 98% can usually be managed with other methods. Further research in San Francisco indicates that only 10% of the 240,000 back surgeries done every year in the U.S. are necessary. Patients should be aware that a doctor specializing in surgery is more likely to treat the ailment surgically than in any other way. Most insurance companies now require second opinions for such surgeries. Make sure you seek other opinions.

Be very cognizant of this time factor: six months is a prudent waiting period from the onset of severe symptoms to actual surgery. However, there are situations when surgery should be done quickly. Watch your pain! If it is excruciating and persistent without relief, if there is also a substantial loss of reflex action or muscle weakness; if there is numbness or impairment of basic bodily functions, (such as problems urinating or defecating); then surgery is necessary, and in fact, should be done without delay. This surgical emergency is called the *cauda equina syndrome* and waiting even 12 hours to treat it is too long.

If you have already had unsuccessful surgery for a bad back, you have joined a large group of people in the failed back surgery syndrome classification. Many of these people have a sacroiliac or facet syndrome. Don't despair! See a chiropractor or an osteopath who does manipulation and get the mechanical dysfunction corrected. If these failed back surgery syndrome patients had recognized that their so-called disc herniation was not necessarily so, they undoubtedly would have taken a different approach.

Of course, some failed back surgeries result from surgeon error or poor healing with too many adhesions. However, after surgery, it is extremely important to make sure the mechanical causes are attended to, so that the surgical repair is not put under the same harmful stresses which caused the need for surgery.

Neurologists

The nerve specialist will determine whether there is damage occurring to the nerves, which causes muscle wasting and weakness. It often happens that by the time the neurologist is consulted, surgery is already inevitable. The disc herniation, like a space-occupying tumor, must be removed. However, it is my experience that many borderline cases are less likely to be sent to a surgeon by a neurologist. Neurologists are more conservative than orthopedists and reserve surgery only for severe disc syndrome cases.

Many back pain professionals believe that if surgery is necessary, a neurologist should perform it. Neurosurgeons are best at handling the delicate intricacies of the spinal nerves.

There may be some controversy here, especially among the orthopedic surgeons. The point is not to let an orthopedist do disc surgery unless you have had a second opinion from a neurologist or neurosurgeon. Remember, there is no hurry unless you are unable to urinate. A few extra days will not cause any permanent damage.

Do not get railroaded into unnecessary surgery. The neurosurgeon will be less likely to misinform you about a small disc bulge seen on an M.R.I. or C.T. scan. Even people who never get back pain can have these small disc bulges.

If your doctor doesn't like the suggestion of your getting a second opinion, then switch doctors! Be wary of back surgery, because it has a very high failure rate.

The Physiotherapists

These specialists usually practice in conjunction with a family practitioner, orthopedist or neurologist. Thus, the physiotherapists are usually the given "prescription" for treatment by the supervising physician. Whenever a decision has to be made about changing a treatment in any way, that decision is normally made by the physician in charge. The physiotherapist then applies the directive to the patient. Since physiotherapists often treat large groups of people, progress with or relief from a particular back problem is not usually measured on a per-visit schedule. Rather, the patient's progress is monitored carefully every 10 visits or so when the patient sees the supervising physician for a follow-up visit.

Recently, however, the traditional role of the physiotherapist has begun to change. More and more, we see these practitioners working independently from physicians, directly managing the patient's treatment from their own points of view.

In some states the physiotherapist is a prime contact practitioner. This means they do not have to work under the supervision of a medical doctor at all, but can make decisions about treatment entirely on their own. In this case, you should be aware that the physiotherapist is in reality doing a medical examination.

In this capacity, they should be conducting tests such as those described in Chapter Two to determine whether the patient has a mechanical dysfunction, or whether he or she has systemic back pain and needs to be referred to a specialist.

• • •

For your own protection, not to mention peace of mind, here is a list of questions that you need to ask your physiotherapist to see if the proper decisions are being made:

1. Have the appropriate tests been completed to diagnose my type of back pain? What is my working diagnosis?

2. Does my back pain have a systemic cause?

If the answer is YES, more than physiotherapy should be employed to gain relief. You should be under a specialist's prescription. You are probably in a stress-distress situation and you need more than reductionistic care, which may be reducing pain and discomfort, but not addressing the specific cause. You may need to consult a clinical psychologist as well as other specialists.

3. If you have mechanical causes of back pain, what are they:

— Locked back joints?
— Shortened muscle groups?
— Locked sacroiliac joints?
— Decreased hip function?
— Pronated ankle (collapsing inward), poor posture, etc.?

4. Is my treatment getting at the causes of my pain as well as reducing the inflammation?

5. How are these underlying causes being monitored?

6. Why am I getting heat for inflammation? (It may feel good at the time, but it encourages swelling.)

7. Can I get modern electrotherapy to reduce inflammation and swelling? (Some physiotherapists may use ice packs for 10 to 12 minutes.)

8. When my pain goes, will you teach me correct posture and exercises to prevent the mechanical problems of shortened muscles, shortened ligaments and joint locking?

If you discover that your treatment is just relieving the pain and not treating the underlying causes, change doctors and therapists. Otherwise, you will only get rid of your back pain temporarily.

Studies have shown that many of the therapy methods used by physiotherapists have absolutely no redeeming effect in the treatment of back pain. For example, it is very difficult to produce evidence that the application of ultrasound is better than doing nothing at all.

If your back has locked joints, or your sacroiliac and hip joints need a manipulation, you should consult a chiropractor or an osteopath. Heat and exercise will not correct the cause of your back pain. Remember, back pain is only a small part of a physiotherapist's training. Post-operative rehabilitation, stroke care and many other hospital conditions are their main concerns.

Rheumatologists

Rheumatoid arthritis is the single largest crippling disease in North America, and one of the chief culprits of chronic joint pain. Rheumatologists specialize in arthritic musculoskeletal diseases. They order specific blood tests and other procedures to arrive at a diagnosis.

Rheumatologists are often consulted when other professional care has not solved the problem by mechanical means. A condition called ankylosing spondylitis, described in Chapter One, is often missed or misdiagnosed when it causes back pain in early adulthood. When these young people do not improve with most treatments, good back specialists should recognize the need for a rheumatologist's opinion. In turn, a good rheumatologist should recognize the high incidence of psychological factors in a rheumatoid patient. Clinical psychologists should also be consulted to determine the cause of the harmful distress in these patients.

Painful muscle conditions called *fibrositis* or *fibromyalgia* (irritations of the muscle fibers) have been linked to insufficient deep sleep. Once again, the rheumatologist can do the necessary diagnostic procedures to uncover the causes of this problem.

You probably need to see a rheumatologist if you get temporary relief from aspirin or some other pain reliever, and/or your condition worsens if treated by any of the more aggressive physio- and manipulative therapies.

Chiropractors

Back pain conditions are the most common complaints seen in a chiropractor's office. Manipulation is the main therapy, along with the use of physical therapy.

For descriptive purposes, chiropractors often tell their patients the cause of back pain is spinal misalignment. They talk about bones being "out," and nerves being "pinched." These are misnomers, as is the term "slipped disc." Discs don't slip and most back pain is not caused by a bone being out of place. The fact is, manipulation changes the mechanics of the joints, and with repetition, establishes correct nerve, muscle, and joint function.

Chiropractors deal with the mechanical group of back disorders, and refer bone cancer and other systemic conditions to other specialists. If you answered yes to one of the questions in the first diagnosis group, you could go to a chiropractor, but most likely you would be referred to another specialist after the diagnostic work-up. On the other hand, if you are suffering from a disc, back joint, sacroiliac joint or muscular-related back pain, you should see a chiropractor.

Research has shown that a very small percentage of disc cases actually need surgery. Two separate studies comparing chiropractic manipulation to hospital outpatient treatment confirmed chiropractic procedures are safe and most effective for nonsurgical back conditions.

To ensure that your chiropractor is up-to-date and practicing modern concepts, a list of questions follows. The information enclosed in parentheses gives the underlying reasons for asking the question.

1. Will you conduct tests to rule out a systemic cause of my back pain?

2. Will you take x-rays no bigger than 14" x 17", and do you use rare earth screens and fast film? (These three factors will reduce your exposure to radiation by 75%. Don't allow a full-spine x-ray to be taken unless *scoliosis* [severe curvature] is suspected.) Will the films be sent to a chiropractic or medical radiologist for a written report? (It will cost more, but it's worth it. This will assure that the film quality is good, and that a bone pathology is not overlooked.)

3. Will you be trying to correct misalignments? Or, will you be restoring mechanical function to my joints? (Manipulation has little effect on realigning the spine. Manipulation does restore range of motion and joint function.)

4. Do you treat and restore function when necessary to my sacroiliacs, hips, knees and ankles for lower back pain? (Do not accept treatment to only your lower back. The cause of pain is rarely only there.)

5. What is your diagnosis? (At this point, remember the four types of mechanical causes. Don't accept the cause as a "misaligned bone pinching a nerve." A pinched nerve radiates pain down from your back and causes tingling or numbness. Check the diagnosis you are given against the test questions in Chapter Two. If you have numbness and muscle weakness, etc., your chiropractor should be ordering special tests and consulting with other specialists to make sure that surgery is not necessary.)

6. After my pain subsides, will you restore normal function to my spine, hips and legs? Will you give me strengthening exercises to prevent further attacks? Your chiropractor should do both.

7. If I have degenerative discs and unstable motion units, will I be provided with regular monthly care to assure that joint locking and muscle spasms are not developing? (Prevention and spinal management are important chiropractic services.)

8. If I am placed under maintenance care on a monthly basis, will you be testing me for: decreased ranges of motion, shortened muscle groups and poor posture? Also, can I get a pre-

scribed home care program to stretch and strengthen my legs and back?

9. What is the therapy for the inflammation, and what part of the treatment is working toward restoring spinal function? (Manipulation should be given where the joints are locked, not necessarily at the point where your back hurts. Physical therapy, such as electrotherapy, applied at the painful, inflamed areas speeds up the recovery. Manipulation of the inflamed area can keep it sore and inflamed. Ask your chiropractor if you are getting more motion in the locked joints. It is not uncommon to need different adjustments or manipulation in different areas of the spine or extremities to get your spine back to normal.)

Massage Therapists

Licensed masseurs/masseuses normally work in cooperation with other practitioners as part of an overall back pain management program. Massage is especially helpful in the treatment of muscle spasms, and also works well if the cause of the backache is a soft-tissue muscle problem.

Massage offers both physiological and psychological benefits. Therapists can ease or prevent muscle spasms, stimulate blood circulation and offer soothing, calming effects by stroking the surface of the body. A therapeutic massage is often effective in speeding up the recovery from muscle pain.

There are sub-groups within this category of specialists, and almost as many techniques as technicians. Basic to all techniques, is that the muscle is manipulated sideways to separate the fibers, or stripped length-wise to elongate the muscle cells. The purpose is to milk toxic acid by-products from the muscle, sending them into general circulation, so the blood can be detoxified by the kidneys and liver. Although this type of massage can be painful, it is beneficial in stretching and lengthening the muscles. Painful muscle trigger-points are also stretched and pressed upon during a therapeutic massage.

Some massage therapists practice a ritualistic procedure requiring one-hour treatments, repeated 10 or 15 times. In these sessions, much of the time is often spent on areas unrelated to your back pain. However, therapeutic massage can reverse the chronic changes in muscles that are frequently the main causal factors in back pain. A general routine massage is usually not sufficient.

If you are considering going to a massage therapist, it is important that you determine whether your condition will respond to the therapy, or whether a co-treatment would be most effective. Massage therapy marries perfectly with chiropractic and osteopathic manipulation, and should be part of any physical therapy approach to back pain.

Osteopaths

There are two different schools of osteopathy. The first is the more traditional approach, wherein the osteopath is a specialist in manipulation and can determine the different causes of back pain. The second type is the modern osteopath. Usually, this person is the equivalent of a medical doctor who has received limited but specialized training in manipulation techniques, and therefore can offer treatments combining drugs, surgery and a limited version of the traditional manipulation therapy.

Back pain patients should seek the osteopathic practitioner using conservative methods, but which do not duplicate the treatments of a medical doctor. Some osteopaths use muscle energy and cranial pressure techniques that are more esoteric. Once again, be sure your mechanical problems are receiving attention. Here is a list of pertinent questions you should ask an osteopath:

1. Are you primarily practicing osteopathic manipulation, with drugs and surgery as a back-up? Will I receive skilled manipulation?

2. Have sufficient tests been conducted to rule out systemic causes?

3. Were x-rays taken and read by an osteopathic, chiropractic or medical radiologist? (Remember, paying a little more for such a service is well worth the price.)

4. What is my diagnosis?

5. How will the inflammation be treated? How will the mechanical problems be treated?

6. Once the pain goes away, what home prevention program will be organized?

7. If you don't do manipulation on a regular basis, can you recommend a practitioner to restore normal function to the locked joints?

Acupuncturists

These practitioners work on the theory that back pain is caused by an imbalance in the body's meridian system. Meridian lines have been charted on the body by ancient Chinese practitioners to illustrate acupuncture points.

After finding something amiss in the patient's meridian points, the acupuncturist places needles along these points in order to balance and normalize the energy. This treatment can often be very effective. Research has found that when these needles are applied, endorphins are produced. *Endorphins* are hormones produced by the brain which have a painkilling effect.

As the pain is relieved, the back sufferer can attain a much better range of motion, which in turn can break the vicious spasm-pain-muscle spasm cycle. This occurs not because the meridians have been balanced, but because the pain has been arrested via the production of endorphins.

The above is a very simplistic explanation of how the acupuncturist can help treat bad backs. Sufferers must be aware that there are many causes of back pain, and they must recognize that many causes would not respond to acupuncture in the long run. Perhaps the pain pattern will respond in some instances, but the underlying cause would remain, and the pain would return.

The field of acupuncture is cluttered with poorly-trained, inexperienced, over-zealous practitioners. Neither a few weekends nor a few hundred hours is long enough for a person to become a specialist. If you seek an acupuncturist make sure that they are adequately qualified.

Remember, too, that for long-lasting relief, the poor mechanics must be corrected. It is not enough just to treat the pain symptoms. If the acupuncture does not lengthen your hamstring muscles or free up a locked sacroiliac joint, for example, you are destined for another back pain episode.

Podiatrists

If your back pain originates in the legs or feet, then this specialist may be able to successfully treat the condition by placing an orthotic device inside your shoe. Specifically, if you have a "sloping in" of the ankle, which is called pronation and is a mechanical cause of back pain, a podiatrist can help with an orthotic, thus taking the torque off your lower back.

Pronation causes the knee and upper leg to rotate forward and inward as well. This forward rotation also carries the pelvis forward on the same side. Walking around with this problem produces a mechanical insult every time the opposite swinging leg tries to rotate the pelvis forward. An average person takes 20,000 to 30,000 of these steps every day. This mechanical stress wears away on your lower back, like the Colorado River gouging out the Grand Canyon.

Informed back pain sufferers should be able to determine if they are candidates for orthotics through their own self-examinations. Otherwise, it would be ridiculous, costly and perhaps even detrimental for a patient to wear orthotics if there were no existing condition to justify it. Remember, to determine whether there is pronation, look at your ankles from behind. Each Achilles tendon should be perpendicular to the floor. The tendon's ridge at the back of your ankle should be straight up from the floor — not angling inwards or outwards.

Temporary orthotics, or bandaging of the affected area, can often determine whether a patient will respond to this type of treatment, thereby avoiding the unnecessary costs of a useless permanent appliance, which can run as high as $1,200. You should never pay more than $400, and many excellent orthotics are available for $175 or less from skilled fitters.

Ask your back specialist to confirm if you have ankle pronation and then have a podiatrist fit you with orthotics.

Allergists

Sometimes back pain is caused by an adverse reaction to a particular food or beverage. It's not completely understood how allergies can manifest themselves as back pain, joint pain or the stiffening of the musculature, but they do. Fortunately, there are ways to determine whether an allergy is the cause or not.

One such way is a four-day fast, undertaken, of course, with the doctor's supervision. During this fast, the patient drinks only water or a bit of fruit juice (hopefully a type he's not allergic to). The water fast removes all the food allergies from the system; quite often by the fourth day, all the aches and pains are also gone! In this way you can determine whether or not you are suffering from back pain caused by an allergic reaction. Unfortunately, in most cases a fast will not help a back pain sufferer.

If the pain is caused by an allergy, then the allergist will know what to do. Coffee is a common culprit for many people suffering from tension and muscle spasm in the mid-back.

We suggest this four-day fast be supervised by a health professional. If the four-day fast clears up your back pain, make an appointment with an allergist.

Nutritionists

These professionals treat lower back pain by determining whether a particular nutrient deficiency or combination thereof is the cause. Lack of nutrients, especially vitamin C or iron, can increase the inflammation in the lower back area. However, you should systematically eliminate any and all possible mechanical causes of your pain before seeking help from a nutritionist. At this time there is little research to support the claim that nutritional supplementation can relieve back trouble.

Many back specialists other than nutritionists recommend vitamin C, multiple minerals and other specific supplements. The rationale is to provide an anti-inflammatory effect and also supply the nutrients needed for healthy, soft tissues. Some supplements are anti-spasmodic and relax the muscles.

I have seen patients who were distressed, malnourished and depleted of nutrients because of smoking or drug use who were definitely helped by nutritional supplements.

If you don't seem to heal as fast as you used to, buy some quality multiple vitamin and mineral tablets and take them as directed for a few months. It can take the body a long time to make up for some nutrient deficiencies.

Psychiatrists / Psychologists

When anxiety amplifies the magnitude of the pain, or when there is any other type of psychological component to the sufferer's back problem, then the patient should be receiving counseling from a psychiatrist or psychologist. This counseling is most effective when done in conjunction with treatment from a back specialist.

When the stress is self-inflicted you can correct the situation yourself. If the causes of your stress and anxiety are not apparent, then you may need professional help. Ask your prime practitioner to refer you to a capable psychotherapist.

It's been known for many years that people who are unhappy with their jobs suffer from back pain and are much more difficult to help than those who are happy at work. It has been shown that patients with a high degree of job satisfaction overcome their back injuries and surgeries better and faster than those who are unhappy with their vocations. Back pain can cause reactive depression which almost always disappears when the pain goes away. However, chronic depression or anxiety can impede or make a full recovery unobtainable.

A good clinical psychologist can do a psychological survey and let you and your back specialist know if a quick recovery is possible without psychological counseling.

Other Techniques and Therapies

Yoga

Most back exercises prescribed by specialists are derived from yoga. Body movement involves muscle strength, muscle and other soft tissue flexibility, physical endurance and balance. Nautilus® and other exercise machines increase muscle strength and endurance. Stretching exercises elongate muscles and increase the elasticity of soft tissue. But yoga does it all, improving strength, endurance, flexibility and balance. The reason that exercises and balancing postures are performed upright with bare feet and sometimes upside down is to impose a demand on the automatically controlled (not consciously-controlled) postural muscles. Yoga also offers a serenity and philosophy that controls stress and promotes a natural, healthful lifestyle.

Many yoga postures create leverages which can cause spontaneous joint manipulation. I personally advise that a skilled motion manipulator should find the joint blockages and correct them before yoga is started. The problem with spontaneous manipulations is that they often cause an adjustment at the inflamed and already mobile joint.

This is why so many experienced yoga masters work with a competent doctor who performs the specific manipulation. The reverse is also true. Once the patient has achieved a mobile, pain-free spine, the doctor should recommend the patient work to achieve strong, flexible muscles and ligaments, as well as to activate the balancing responses. Yoga is a wonderful method of achieving these desired results.

Temporomandibular Joint (TMJ) Therapy

This controversial procedure involves treating back pain by the placing of dental splints in the mouth. The theory behind it holds that the TMJ problem causes muscular imbalance in the lower back. TMJ therapy is both a highly expensive and possibly dangerous approach which should be viewed with a great deal of skepticism, especially since dentists are not in agreement.

It is imperative that all other possible causes of back pain have been fully examined and discounted before starting this precarious and controversial form of therapy. Not only will it ultimately cost thousands of dollars to try this method, but I suggest that this is a minor cause of back pain problems. It's a very remote possibility that your back pain originates in the mouth.

There should be a psychological assessment completed by a clinical psychologist to assure the back pain is not predominantly part of a neurosis. Obviously, this test would commence at the conclusion of failed correction of the mechanical dysfunction by a previous professional and proper self-help exercises and stretches.

My advice is to be sure you are a very well informed consumer before you sign up for expensive and questionable TMJ therapy. Those rare few patients who need their temporo-mandibular joint function restored will respond to TMJ manipulation and TMJ muscle-stretching techniques. If these procedures only give temporary relief, a permanent splint or dental work may be necessary for lasting success.

Back School

Back schools consist of about four or five lectures and workshops dedicated to removing the anxiety, thereby reducing the stress, of back pain. The schools also teach good posture, exercises and basic movements of sitting, lifting, walking and sleeping.

Recent research has shown that back schools are achieving high marks for good results. In many instances these results are as good as those obtained by other health professionals who deal directly with the treatment of back pain. This proves you don't always need direct treatment.

Back school usually starts after or during a successful treatment plan and should combine the best of all the therapies. After seeing the fine results from back school, orthopedists, chiropractors and physiotherapists are developing a multi-disciplinary program for the schools.

Patients who attend these schools receive the necessary information applicable to changing bad habits and lifestyles that have been major causes of their back pain. The average cost for back school is normally between $80 to $100.

The success rate is getting so high that insurance companies are beginning to pay for back school attendance. The schools are especially helpful as a follow-up after a series of treatments has set you free from pain.

Because the programs teach workers how to avoid occupational hazards, large corporations and industries now realize it pays to put high-risk employees through these schools.

Hopefully, reading this book will serve as a kind of back school program for you.

•   •   •

Chapter Four

The Therapies

"If it seems ridiculous . . . it probably is."

There are many accepted therapeutic methods to stop back pain. Some are temporary pain relievers. Some remove the causal factors. Still others keep the patient occupied and satisfied as the body heals in spite of the interference.

Drug Therapy

On the surface, this therapy would appear to be the easiest way to get relief from back problems. Unfortunately, drugs treat more than the affected area of pain and carry the risk of side effects which are oftentimes much worse and more debilitating than the original back pain.

Drug therapy is divided into three main groups: 1. The Anti-inflammatories; 2. The Pain Killers, and 3. The Muscle Relaxants. Sometimes an anti-depressant is also prescribed.

Anti-inflammatory Drugs

The anti-inflammatory drugs are steroids (such as cortisone) or non-steroidal (such as ibuprofen, the ingredient in Motrin® and Advil®).

The steroids have the most serious side effects and should not be accepted as treatment without previous therapeutic failures. Their side effects can cause serious demineralization of the bones and fluid retention, which leads to other health problems.

The non-steroidal drugs, such as Motrin® and aspirin, are very effective at reducing inflammation. Yet, some studies show that their use can also depress the healing process. This prolongs the need for continued anti-inflammatory therapy. These drugs should never be used daily on a long-term basis. They do not deal with the cause of the inflammation and they distort the healing process.

The Pain Killers

Pain killers such as aspirin (Bufferin®, Bayer's®) and acetaminophen (Tylenol®) should only be used on a short-term basis. However, the cause of the back pain must always be addressed in order to treat the problem. The theory behind taking pain killers is to deaden the pain enough to allow better joint movement, and hence increase joint function. This, in turn, will stimulate nerve endings, blocking the pain response, and also relax the spastic muscles. The body can then get on with healing itself, especially if the cause of pain is corrected.

The Muscle Relaxants

Muscle relaxants work on much the same theory as the pain killers and the two are often prescribed together. The relaxation of the muscle spasm reduces the pain caused by the spasm and allows freer joint function. Restoring normal function is the primary goal of all back specialists. More practitioners are working together these days. My patients are often prescribed pain killers, non-steroidals, anti-inflammatories and muscle relaxants to help facilitate spinal manipulative therapy.

General practitioners and chiropractors working together can achieve marvelous results. As the patient, you must orchestrate this approach yourself. Most family practitioners are not familiar with modern, rational spinal and extremity joint manipulation. By the same token, most chiropractors are not accustomed to requesting short-term drug therapy to reduce pain and inflammation. If you have two rational doctors to whom you suggest cooperative therapy management, they will undoubtedly like the arrangement. They may even learn to treat other patients the same way if they are not already doing so.

Never be afraid to take matters of your health into your own hands. Doctors take an oath to help the patient foremost. Beware of the doctor who has an ego too big to allow cooperative effort. He's probably just out for monetary gain, at your's and other patients' expense.

Cold Packs

These are the simplest home remedy for anti-inflammatory reduction, muscle relaxation and pain relief. But be forewarned: you should not apply ice on the painful area for more than 15 minutes at a time. Otherwise, the tissue will become too chilled and the body will send more blood to warm up the tissue. Over-chilling encourages swelling by increasing the size of the small blood vessels called capillaries. In essence, it reverses reduction of the swelling and inflammation that the initial cold pack produces. It's better to apply the ice for 10 to 12 minutes, remove it for an hour, and then apply it again for another 10 to 12 minutes. You will find this gives you the best and safest home remedy for anti-inflammatory care.

Electrotherapy

There are many different varieties of electrotherapy, some more effective than others for treating back pain. Electrotherapy utilizes machines to pass a very mild electric current from an electrode pad placed on the surface of the skin. Some currents kill pain, and some reduce swelling and inflammation, while others strengthen weakened muscles. In my experience, the most effective and comfortable machine for doing all of the above is an interferential machine.

Interferential therapy is applied by placing four electrode pads around the area of inflammation in your back. Two mild cross-currents somewhat out of phase with each other create a three dimensional electric field that encompasses the inflamed area. This electric field can be controlled by varying the difference between the two currents. The most effective anti-inflammatory/pain-relieving effects are achieved by currents that prickle the skin as they pass through, but are not strong enough to cause muscle contraction. Each application lasts from 12 to 20 minutes. Anything less will not give the patient the optimum benefit of the treatment, and too much is superfluous.

These mild currents have multiple beneficial effects and replace the need for other electrotherapy that achieves only one specific reaction. A simple physical stimulation of the inflamed area of your back only achieves limited results. The circulation may be increased, the swelling reduced, the pain deadened, the healing process speeded up, and the weakened muscles strengthened, but nothing replaces the overall multiple effects of interferential therapy when properly applied.

Electrotherapy is usually applied daily or every other day for up to 10 applications. In the chronically inflamed back, it could take months to eliminate the inflammation and pain. There are some old and many new electrotherapy units, but the goal remains the same: to produce a physiological effect which promotes your own body's healing process.

Ultrasound

The ultrasound machine uses a very high frequency radio crystal to transmit sound waves through your skin into the painful area of your back. It is my least favorite treatment. Studies have shown it to be almost useless for back pain. And even worse is its potential to cause harm. With sloppy application the sound waves cause an inflammatory reaction to the covering of the bone, which can be quite painful.

If ultrasound has not helped after 10 applications, it never will. Do not let anyone apply it any longer if it has failed to help you recover.

Transcutaneous Electrical Nerve Stimulation (TENS)

This is another form of electrotherapy. It is portable and, at best, acts as a pain reducer or pain killer. You may have tried one or seen someone wearing a small power pack on their belt. The TENS unit is about the size of a small pocket radio with two or four wires attached. The electrodes at the end of the wires are placed near the spine, where a mild current is emitted to block the pain.

You can buy a TENS unit for a few hundred dollars, or rent one. They are easy to use, but the wires can be a nuisance. Their usage should be temporary at most, as some recent studies question their value.

Manipulation

History of the Technique

It appears early man knew almost instinctively that manipulation helped ease back pain. Manipulation of the spine and extremity joints dates back before recorded time. Mayan pottery sculptures depict individuals being stretched and stressed upon. Cave dwellers' art clearly shows people being manipulated, as do the earliest writing tablets.

Around the Sixth Century A.D., manipulation fell into ill repute. A powerful Roman pope of the time decreed that surgery and manipulation were heresy. Surgery was the first of these two techniques to come out of the dark ages, while manipulation got its emancipation in the late 1880s or early 1900s.

A self-educated Canadian by the name of Dan Palmer developed chiropractic. Simultaneously, around 1885, a medical doctor named Andrew Still developed osteopathy. Both chiropractic and osteopathy became full-fledged professions, in spite of heavy medical opposition from the medical community, which included the use of some illegal tactics by medical doctors who felt threatened by the new sciences. In the famous 1989 Wilkes case in Illinois, the American Medical Association (AMA) was found guilty of using illegal tactics against chiropractic. To oppose osteopathic medicine, they absorbed and then distorted the principles.

Recently, in most countries of the world, these old battles have been completely forgotten. The education level of chiropractors has risen so significantly that their research is now being widely published. Here in the U.S., many interdisciplinary societies and conferences continue to develop, and the necessary exchange of important scientific information is occurring.

Rational dialogue and cooperation are leading to better treatment for patients suffering from a multitude of nerve, muscle and bone disorders. Athletes and weekend warriors alike are also finding they can overcome injuries and achieve better performance with the help of manipulation.

How the Technique Works

The joint space is enclosed by a capsular sack containing the joint fluid. This fluid lubricates the slippery surfaces and supplies nutrients in a blood-free zone. Manipulation, or "adjustment," as chiropractors term it, is the physical separation of the joint space. When the joint surfaces are separated by just a few millimeters, the area of the joint space is increased, thus lowering the pressure on the fluids inside the joint.

When your chiropractor performs manipulation, a cracking sound is heard as gases pop out of the joint fluid. This is the same phenomenon as gas bubbles appearing in a bottle of soda when the cap is removed. Once this cavitation has occurred, the joint can glide on this nitrogen gas bubble for 20 minutes as the patient experiences an increase in the range of motion with much less pain.

The most rational approach to manipulation is to adjust the joint with the lost range of motion, not the inflamed joint producing the pain. At a recent interdisciplinary conference where I presented a lecture on the topic, the panel of experts came to the conclusion that manipulation should be used to remove the cause of the mechanical malfunction. Doctors from varied professions confirmed that one cannot and should not manipulate inflamed joints. The skilled chiropractor or osteopath should manipulate the locked joints above, below and opposite the inflamed joint.

Manipulation should be repeated daily or every other day until all ranges of motion are restored. Full recovery of motions is usually achieved after the pain has stopped in the nearby inflamed area of the spine.

Manipulation removes a major cause of back pain, which is the blockage or lack of normal function in a joint that cannot be restored by exercising or stretching. It's a shame so many sufferers are exercising with abnormal function and thus establishing pain-free compensations. These compensations will lead to more serious degenerative complications, as we saw with the aerobics instructor in Chapter One. "Manipulation first and exercise later" is what I always recommend. Used in this sequence, the exercise helps re-establish the normal biomechanics needed for a pain-free back.

Manipulation must not be a war between the forces of the manipulator and the holding elements of a joint. The best manipulation is a pleasant experience as the sense of tension is released.

Occasionally a healing crisis occurs after a manipulation. This is like a fever which peaks right before it breaks — you perspire profusely, and then feel much better. Although this crisis can be painful, most of the pain and inflammation disappears after 24 to 48 hours. Good reactions to a manipulation are a general flood of perspiration over your entire body, and a feeling of warmth. Patients often get very sleepy after the first few treatments. Almost everyone has a great sense of well-being, because the spine feels good when it is loose and mobile.

Experience has shown me that everyone could benefit from having at least two full spine manipulations every year. This can prevent faulty biomechanics from developing. But make sure your doctor is only manipulating the joints he finds locked or blocked. Cracking normal joints is not a good preventative procedure.

Manipulation increases motion, and motion promotes proper healing.

Balancing Exercises

Although gymnastics, yoga and other traditional exercise systems challenge the balance mechanisms, back pain sufferers in general do not participate in such activities to achieve the benefits. Research from former Communist Eastern bloc countries confirms the effectiveness of spending a few minutes each day on rocker and balance boards. These studies reveal that balancing exercises cause marked changes in the function of the important automatically controlled smaller back muscles.

Although these methods have not yet gravitated to the West, it will not be long before back pain specialists and body movement instructors from around the world devise unique and funfilled ways to develop our balance reflexes. The result will be much more lasting rehabilitation from a back attack.

Massage

The back and hip joint muscles of a chronic back pain sufferer deteriorate to a weakened and *fibrotic* state, a process which involves a lessening in the contracting tissue and an increase in the noncontractile tissue. A skilled massage therapist works at separating the fibrotic fibers and improving the circulation in these static muscles.

Degenerated muscle cells and supporting tissue can be regenerated with skilled massage when combined with electrotherapy and exercise programs. Sadly, many massage therapists lack the knowledge and skills to achieve this, and most patients expect too much too soon.

Muscle trigger points should be treated by the doctor, yet for more permanent results the same muscles can be elongated and rehabilitated by massage.

The best situation is for the massage therapist to work under prescription from a doctor. The doctor will determine the degenerative status of the muscle groups and confirm that the massage therapist knows the number of weeks needed to attain adequate muscle tissue response.

Non-therapeutic massage, which can be soothing, superficial, and pleasant, is almost useless for most back pain sufferers. I am not opposed to this sort of treatment for reducing stress, but it is ineffective for dealing with chronic muscle changes.

The good massage therapists are known by the good doctors. Neither professional should try to do the impossible themselves. Most back pain sufferers have a complex set of problems, not just a single cause, and the muscles need attention, especially in chronic cases.

A competent doctor/massage therapist team can achieve a tremendous amount of good for a bad back.

Let the Buyer Beware

There's no need for you to become a classic back pain sufferer. If your doctor becomes upset with you for being an informed consumer of his health care, then go elsewhere because he's bluffing you.

You will not alter this disease process by a single action of one of the following:

- Sticking needles in your back or along the liver meridian.
- Taking pain killers.
- Getting your back tapped by a tiny spring-loaded hammer.
- Lying on a few wedge-shaped blocks.
- Taking anti-inflammatories by pill or injection.
- Meditating daily.
- Applying heat packs and ultrasound.
- Getting back manipulation and/or mobilization.
- Having your cranuim reshaped.
- Having an orthotic device placed in your shoe.
- Wearing a red flannel band around your waist.
- Wearing an orthopedic support belt.
- Avoiding lifting, bending or twisting.
- Hanging upside down daily.
  Etc., etc., etc.

These treatments are useless, unless combined with other treatments, if you want lasting results.

• • •

Chapter Five:

Home Treatment

*"One-third knowledge and inspiration,
one-third perspiration,
and one-third relaxation."*

The most important rule for successful treatment of back pain is to obtain the correct diagnosis. This rule holds true for home as well as professional care. Make sure you understand the previous chapters on self-diagnosis, the specialists and the therapies before you begin treating yourself at home.

Therapeutic Goals of Home Treatment

You will be aiming for several therapeutic goals by home treatment of your back pain.

These include:

- Reducing pain
- Reducing inflammation
- Reducing swelling
- Promoting healing of primary tissue
- Discouraging adhesive scar tissue formation
- Increasing the active and passive ranges of back motion by stretching
- Increasing back strength
- Increasing strength of supportive abdominal and pelvic structures
- Increasing passive ranges of motion in the ligaments
- Improving posture
- Improving lifting methods
- Reducing stress factors
- Reducing the body fat-to-muscle ratio
- Learning an effective relaxation technique.

You should already be sharing many of these goals with your doctor or therapist, and achieving greater results with their help. However, if you can also be carrying out rational, intelligent home care you can help yourself speed up the healing process. Let's examine each of these goals individually:

Reducing Pain

If you feel you have strained or sprained your back, the best remedy is ice. Never use heat! Don't even take a hot shower. If you must, take a quick, lukewarm shower. But be sure to use an ice pack for 10 to 12 minutes every hour, especially for the first several hours.

Place the ice directly over the most painful area. This will restrict the swelling, lessen the pain, reduce the reactive muscle spasm and speed up the overall recovery process. Using ice quickly and consistently as described above is time well spent. Don't ever avoid this step. It is always advisable to use the ice pack for 10 to 12 minutes per hour, repeating hourly as often as possible in the first 24 hours. Do not leave the ice on longer than 12 minutes at a time!

The old remedy of bed rest for strain or sprain has proven to be worse than useless. It actually delays recovery. When you have pain, it is advisable to refrain from normal activity. But be sure to keep varying your postures from lying on one side, to sitting, kneeling, standing, walking, lying on your back with your legs over a chair, to lying face down, etc.

Most over-the-counter pain killers help reduce pain, but they have also been known to interfere with the healing process. Some topical cremes and salves create a cold sensation on the skin to distract you away from pain.

To a small degree, pain can be controlled by a TENS unit which is sometimes prescribed for home use. If you must, get one with a variable electrical output. The body can become accustomed to a constant electrical output level and then the pain-killing effect is lost. If I sound somewhat skeptical it's because I have never seen very good results from the use of a TENS unit.

Reducing Inflammation

Inflammation is the body's response to injury. It is designed to ward off and restrict bacterial infections from gaining access to the bloodstream. This is great, except that in 99.9% of back pain injuries there is no infection to wall off. So the sooner the inflammatory process can be stopped and dissipated, the better.

There are a myriad of prescription and over-the-counter anti-inflammatory drugs and techniques which effectively reduce inflammation. However, the real secret to reducing inflammation is to use an ice pack, which has no side effects.

Reducing Swelling

Swelling should be reduced as soon as possible with ice. Yet, for most back pain sufferers the swelling is not apparent, because it is internal. The main exception is the sacroiliac joints which often swell quite visibly. Use ice packs in the same way described above, and remember not to spare the ice!

Promoting Healing of Primary Tissue

To promote healing of primary tissue, you must supply your body with the nutrients it needs. It is vital to increase your intake of vitamin C, and to eat plenty of fresh fruits and vegetables which will supply the necessary vitamin A and essential minerals. If it is difficult or impossible for you to spend a few minutes in the sunshine, be sure to supplement your diet with vitamin D.

Don't exercise your back if it causes any pain lasting more than a few seconds. Rest promotes healing, but too much bed rest is neither necessary nor advisable. While you are relaxing keep changing your postures. Kneel, sit, stand, stretch, lie face up, face down or on your side. Try to keep yourself from maintaining any one posture for more than 20 minutes.

Traveling entails the same principles of relaxation and varying your positions. If you must drive a long distance, make sure you stop the car and walk around for a few minutes every hour. Likewise, for air travel, make it a point to walk up and down the aisles frequently.

Discouraging Adhesive Scar Tissue Formation

When the pain is no longer acute and you are in the healing process, it is important to isolate movement and stretches at the painful area. Don't let healing occur with a shortened muscle condition.

Your body will repair the tissue by following natural laws. Tissue will be supplied to fulfill the need of the imposed demand. If the demand is movement, then normal and elastic tissue will regenerate. During the state of rest or immobility, adhesions will develop and a second-rate healing job will result.

In my 30 years of practice I have rarely prescribed a lumbar back support. A narrow, flexible trochanteric belt that goes around the hips will amply support the sacroiliac joints and allow more lumbar motion. Dockworkers, long-shoremen and others in heavy-lifting occupations wear these wide leather belts around the outside of their trousers at hip level. When they want to lift something heavy, they simply tighten the belt and thus strengthen the supporting ligaments.

The following pictures and descriptions of very important exercises and stretches are arranged in degrees of increasing difficulty. If your back is presently painful, do the first group only. As your back improves, move on to the second group of exercises.

If your back is pain-free at the moment and you are assured the lower back and pelvic biomechanics are normal or close to normal, then use Groups One and Two as warm-ups for the third group of exercises.

The rule is very simple: Any exercise that causes a lingering pain must be discontinued temporarily. An exercise that only hurts for an instant with no pain afterwards must be continued until it becomes pain-free over time.

These exercises are best performed after a warm-up walk of at least 10 minutes. Follow the instructions under the photograph and do your routine daily.

The body responds to an imposed demand by making a specific adaptation. Each of these exercises and stretches are demanding specific changes to help you remove the shackles of back pain.

Just as you cannot learn to play the piano in a few weeks, you cannot achieve new ranges of motion, muscle coordination, balance and strength in your lower back in a few weeks.

Start out gently and build up over months to a vigorous routine. The worse your condition, the longer it will take. However, if you don't get a little better at first, you can't get a lot better later.

Group One: Increasing the Ranges of Back Motion During Recovery

You can only increase your ranges of motion as your pain subsides. The exercises illustrated in Figures 29 through 39 increase the active ranges. Be sure to read the instructions with each photograph before you attempt these exercises.

Group Two: Increasing Back Strength and Supportive Abdominal and Pelvic Structures

Figures 40, 41 and 42 show the first of the second group of exercises that you should start as soon as your back begins to feel better. If you have a good back, these are done as warm-up stretches to more strenuous exercise or a sports activity. Golfers and tennis players must do these to prevent lower back rotational injuries.

The back strengthening exercises are also described in detail in Figures 42 to 56. Again, read the instructions carefully, and follow them exactly for best results.

Group Three: Increasing Ranges of Motion When Fully Recovered

Stretching is the ultimate home care procedure for real long-term benefit. The muscles and ligaments need not only become stronger, they must become more flexible. No matter how many years have passed since you could bend and twist easily, you can and must do it again. A repeated demand for elongation exerted upon each muscle group for at least 30 seconds every day will show you amazing results.

This group of stretches constitutes the warm-up and prevention series. They should be performed daily or before any sports or heavy work activity. If you have worked your way through the first two groups, Figures 57 through 62 will be easily achieved.

Figure 25 and Figure 27 from earlier in the book are additional strenuous exercises that should be included when your strength has increased and you are pain-free.

Improving Posture

It is worth striving for good posture. The best standing posture is that point where you can raise up onto your toes without first having to rock forward. (Remember the example of this in Figure 13 from the Self-Diagnosis chapter?) Starting at your ear lobe, someone should be able to drop an imaginary straight line bisecting your shoulder, and passing just in front of your ankle bone. While sitting, do not slump forward

continued on page 117

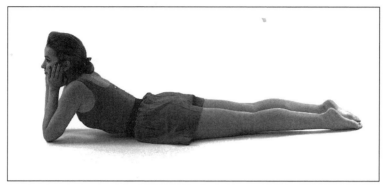

Fig. 29

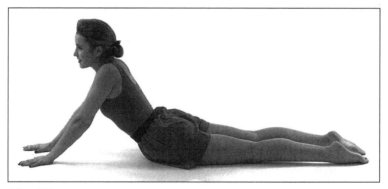

Fig. 30

You should be able to lie as shown in Figure 29, completely relaxed, for 15 minutes. If you have a disc syndrome, it will be necessary to start with a few minutes each day. Do not do the straight arm version (Figure 30) until you can do 15 minutes of the bent-elbow version without causing any pain. In the beginning, these postures may make it very difficult for you to get up off the floor because of a locked feeling. First lower yourself down to a flat position, roll over on your side, kneel, and then get up.

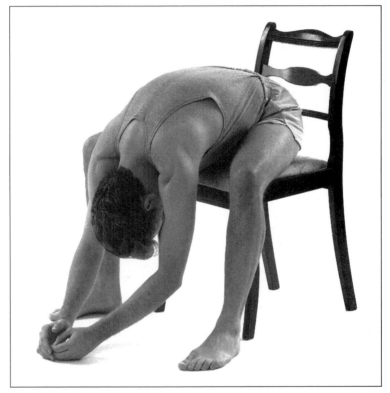

Fig. 31

If you have an active disc syndrome, this position will be difficult for you. Just lean forward to the point of pain and try to relax into the pain very slightly. If it causes you a lingering pain, stop this stretch; if not, increase the forward bend a little each day. With most other back pains, this position will feel good and you can gradually work towards a full relaxed lumbar and hip flexion.

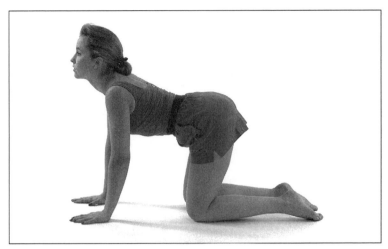

Fig. 32

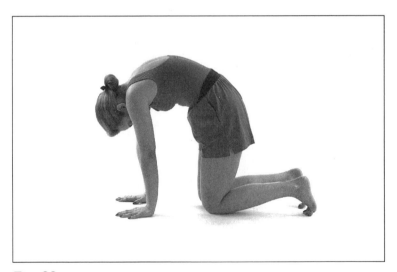

Fig. 33

First let your lower back sag, as in figure 32, to increase the hollow of the lumbar spine while you exhale. Inhale and raise your back like a scared cat on the backyard fence, as in Figure 33. Exhale and let your back sag as far into the hollow as possible. Hold each posture for a few seconds. If it does not hurt, gently sway your hips from side to side while raising and lowering your back.

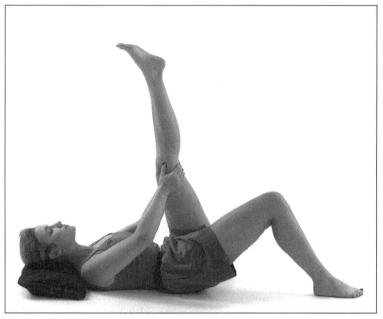

Fig. 34

This is the easiest way to start stretching the hamstring muscles at the back of your thigh. To produce a greater stretch, first contract the hamstrings isometrically, then release. Repeat three times. To take the tension off your lower back, keep your relaxed leg bent with that foot flat on the floor. Raise the leg to be stretched, keeping your knee straight. Hold the back of your knee with your hands so you can resist trying to lower your leg to the floor. Hold this effort and resistance for the count of sixteen and then actively raise your straight leg higher, pulling gently with your hands.

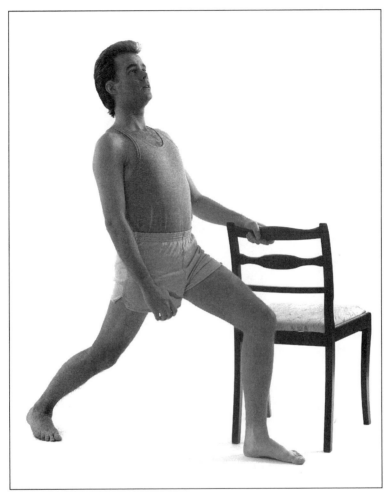

Fig. 35

As with all stretches, hold this one for 30 seconds and exhale for the last five seconds of the stretch. A stretch should not be painful, just a little uncomfortable. As you get better, you can stretch the large hip flexor muscle that attaches to the lower spine even more effectively by turning the back foot inwards and bending the forward knee more than shown.

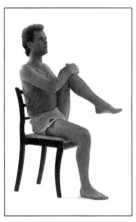 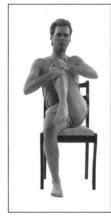 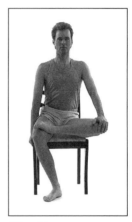

Fig. 36   Fig. 37   Fig. 38

These three hip and sacroiliac stretches have helped more back pain sufferers than any other home care I have ever recommended. Hold each stretch for 30 seconds and do both legs. You must keep your back upright for all of these stretches. Figure 36 is a pull straight up to the shoulder on the same side. Notice the hands clasp the knee, not the lower leg. Figure 37 is a pull to the opposite shoulder for 30 seconds. Finally you push down on your knee for 30 seconds, as in Figure 38.

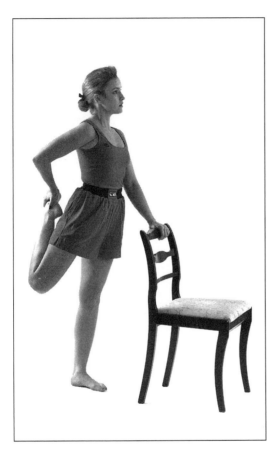

This simple stretch is very effective for the muscles on the front of the thigh. Stand upright and hold the stretch on each side for 30 seconds. Once you can pull your heel so it easily touches your buttock, add more stretch by moving your knee backwards.

Fig. 39

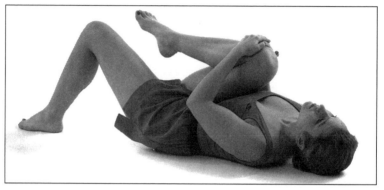

Fig. 40

Pulling one knee up to your chest should be painless before you progress to pulling both knees up to your chest. Make sure you clasp your knees and not your lower leg. Clasping your lower leg increases the leverage on the knee joint and causes too much forced flexion. If you have no pain while pulling both knees toward you, you can then increase the stretch to your lower back by lifting your head off the floor.

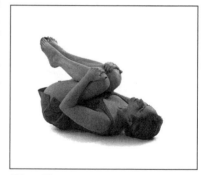

Fig. 41

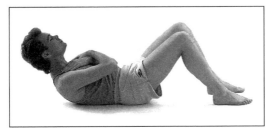

Fig. 42

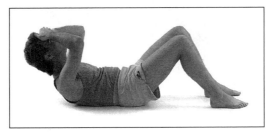

Fig. 43

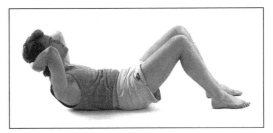

Fig. 44

Make sure your back and feet are flat on the floor as Figure 42 shows. Lift your head, neck and shoulders off the floor for a count of eight and slowly lower back, shoulders and head to the floor to a count of four. When you can easily repeat this exercise 10 times, place your hands on your forehead, as shown in Figure 43, and proceed with the sit-ups as described above. The most strenuous sit-up you can do when your back is recovering is with your hands behind your neck (Figure 44). However, make sure in this position that you do not pull your neck forward with your arms.

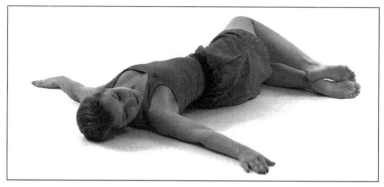

Fig. 45

This is a relaxing rotational stretch. Exhale as you turn your head to the opposite side of your legs. Slowly reverse sides and breath out and relax your lower back again. Repeat from side to side 10 times. Do not do this quickly until your back is fully pain-free.

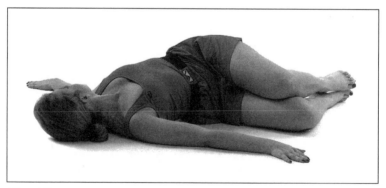

Fig. 46

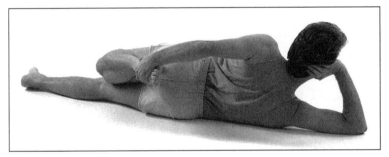

Fig. 47

If holding this stretch for 30 seconds is far too easy, bring your knee back behind the straight leg as far as you can without causing pain on the front of your thigh.

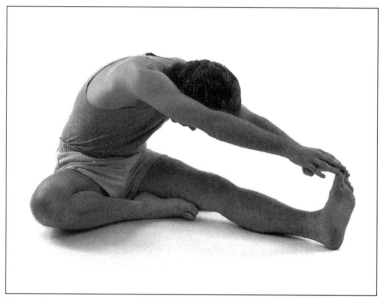

Fig. 48

This hamstring stretch is not harmful when you are recovering because one knee is fully bent. Hold this position for 30 seconds and breathe out for the last five seconds. As you exhale and relax forward, clasp your leg with your hands as far down as you can and hold for another 30 seconds. At first, you may only be able to touch just below your knee. Do not bounce up and down. Bouncing will shorten instead of lengthen the muscle.

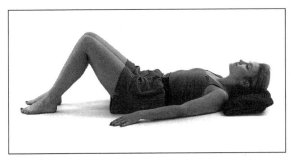

Fig. 49

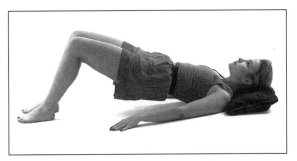

Fig. 50

*Place your feet flat on the floor about a foot apart. Lift your
buttocks as high as you can from the floor and hold for a
count of eight, then gradually lower back to the floor to the
count of four. Build up until you can repeat this 10 times
without pain. Between each lift, push your lower back into
the floor for a count of five. This will strengthen the two
muscle groups that rock your pelvis.*

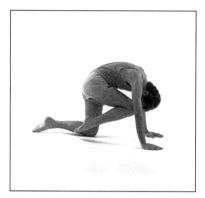

Fig. 51

Start this exercise by repeating the action of bringing your knee up to your shoulder and then straightening your leg out behind you. If this action is easy, hold your leg out behind you for the count of eight. Repeat the sequence 10 times for each leg. For further strengthening, raise the opposite arm, as in Figure 53.

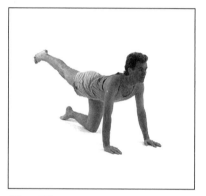

Fig. 52

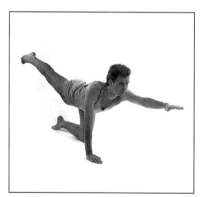

Fig. 53

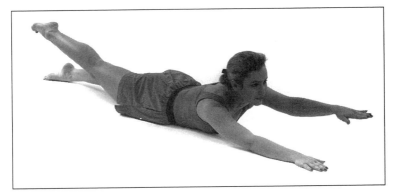

Fig. 54

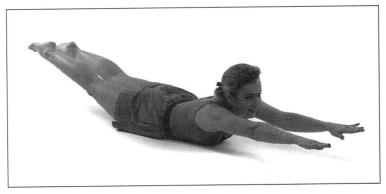

Fig. 55

Hold the opposite arm and leg up as high as you can for a count of eight and lower slowly. Reverse arms and legs and repeat four times. Raise both arms and legs at the same time and hold for a count of eight. When this becomes easy to perform actively, cross your legs above and below each other in a scissors movement eight times as you hold both arms out in front.

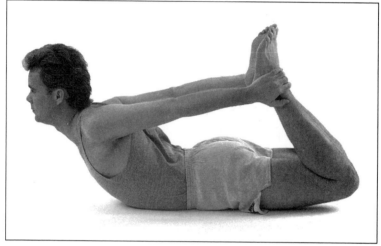

Fig. 56

Once you have raised your head and chest off the ground, separate your knees and raise them off the ground as well. Hold this action for the count of eight. Repeat four times.

into a C shape. Keep the hollow in your lower back. Sit on your thighs, not your tail bone.

It's easy to fall into bad habits, but it's worth practicing the correct ones until they become second nature. The best, and some say the only, way to change posture, is by way of your balance mechanisms.

Posture muscles are controlled by involuntary nerves, which are not influenced by voluntary muscle action. The act of balancing occurs too quickly for conscious correction. Posture is an involuntary action which must be challenged by our balance mechanism action. Try exercising in your bare feet and spend a little time walking with a book balanced on your head. Yoga balancing exercises are extremely beneficial. Some therapists and doctors are beginning to use rockers and balance boards to awaken and change established muscle patterns.

Improving Lifting Methods

Never, never lift anything, not even a pencil or piece of paper, with your knees straight. And don't even think of bending over with straight legs to pick something up and then bending your knees afterwards. If you violate either of these rules, you're asking for, and will probably get, trouble in the form of back pain.

The correct way to lift is to bend your knees first and then bend forward from the hips and waist. Square up to the object you are going to lift so you are never twisted to one side or the other. If the object is even slightly heavy, exhale as you lift. If the object is really heavy, give a

continued on page 119

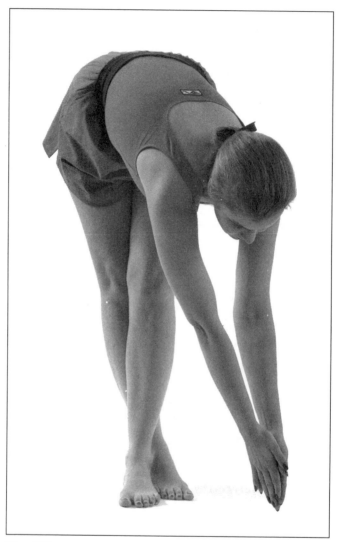

Fig. 57

This is a great hamstring stretch for the back of the leg. Obviously, it has to be repeated in reverse to stretch the other leg. The danger with this stretch is in returning to an upright position. Be sure to unlock your knees and bend them slightly before you rise to an upright position.

good grunt, like professional weight-lifters do. This exhaling allows the release of interdiscal pressure.

Heavy lifting is an acquired skill. Never lift heavy objects on an occasional basis, because your muscles and ligaments need to be hardened for lifting. Think before you try to lift something which may be too heavy for you. If you still get the urge to "give it a try," lie down until the urge passes, or better yet, get someone to help you lift it.

If you have an occupation requiring a lot of bending, stooping and an overall strong back, then you need to spend at least 15 minutes stretching and warming up before you start work. Smart employers will allow this preparation on company time. It'll save them more money in the long run over the inflated insurance premiums and increased workers compensation payments when too many injury claims are filed.

Most sprains and strains occur early in the work day. This is because cold muscles and tight tendons and ligaments sustain injury more easily than warm ones. Do the exercises and stretches recommended in this book. If you have a job loading and unloading trucks, always warm up before you load or unload, especially if you've been driving for an hour or more.

Reducing the Stress Factors

Reducing stress and learning an effective relaxation method go hand-in-hand. It is well known that people unhappy with their jobs are

continued on page 124

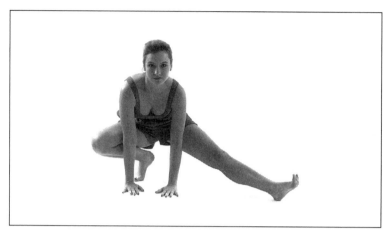

Fig. 58

This is a stretch for the groin muscles and should not be performed if you have pain in your bent knee. Don't bounce. Relax into a good 30-second stretch. The further your foot is out to the side, the more stretch you obtain. Go slowly and be careful.

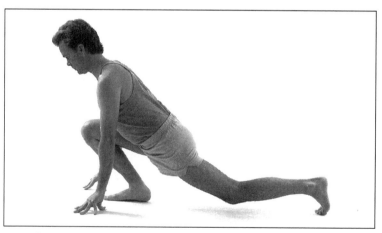

Fig. 59

This is a better stretch if you turn your back foot inwards a few degrees. If your front knee cannot take the stress, kneel on the forward leg rather than having your foot flat on the floor. Don't forget to hold all stretches for 30 seconds and exhale during the last five seconds.

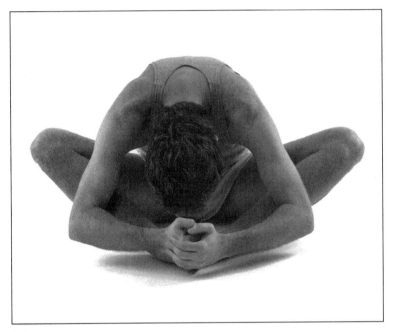

Fig. 60

This is the ultimate back flexing and hip stretching exercise. It can take most back sufferers almost a year of daily stretches to achieve this level of flexibility. While sitting on the floor, place the soles of your feet together with legs bent. Slowly try to bring your upper body, led by your head, downward towards your feet. The objective is to place your head as close as possible to your feet.

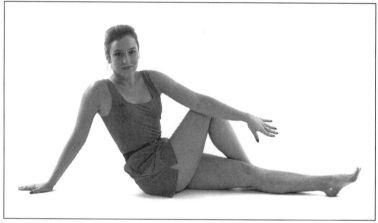

Fig. 61

Relax your lower back; however, at the same time push with your arm against your knee to achieve more rotation. There should be a good stretch of your buttock on the bent leg and your lower back. Hold for 30 seconds, then exhale for more rotation. Hold the gain with your arm and relax your lower back even more. Then repeat with the other leg.

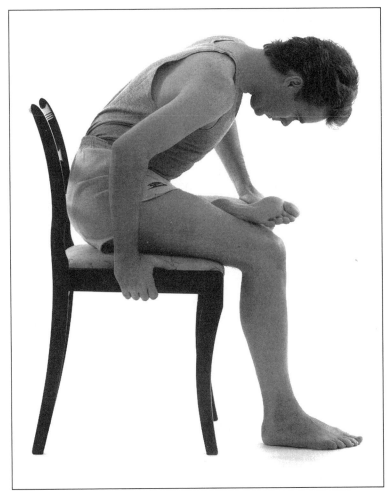

Fig. 62

This exercise stretches the short, powerful hip rotators in your buttocks. In the second group of exercises we did not lean forward. But in this exercise, the further you lean forward, the better the stretch. Be careful when returning to an upright position. Push back up with your arms before you use your back muscles. After this exercise, stand up and lean backwards, with your hands supporting your low back. Hold this counter-stretch for a count of eight.

much more likely to make slow recoveries from back pain than those who are highly motivated to go to work. Thus, job satisfaction is most important in reducing stress.

However, if you can't escape the stress, then it is imperative for you to learn an effective, relaxation and stress-reducing technique. As you shall see, Chapter Six is devoted entirely to a time-proven, well-tested method of relaxation which I have been prescribing for years.

Many types of meditation shift the body out of the harmful "fight-or-flight" syndrome and into the calm side of the nervous system. These methods do work. They promote a healing response and offer a sense of security. The act of visualization has also been reported by surgeons to positively influence healing.

Aerobic Exercise and Reducing the Body Fat-to-Muscle Ratio

Being overweight may not be healthy, but no one has ever proven that it increases the incidence of back pain. However, it is my experience that losing weight helps clear up back pain. Maybe the exercise needed to shed poundage is the rational reason for the decrease in lower back pain.

Always walk at least three times a week. As your back pain subsides, begin walking for ever-increasing periods of time up to a minimum maintenance time of 40 minutes. If your location is not conducive to an outdoor, early morning fresh air walk, then get access to a motorized treadmill. When walking, swing your arms and take good-sized steps. Small steps will not sufficiently extend the hip joints or demand enough pelvic action.

While fast walking does not cause back pain, you should definitely hold off on jogging until you are free of pain. Being a doctor who walks but does not jog, I never encourage people to jog for aerobic conditioning. The benefits of walking vs. jogging could fill another volume, so I will say no more.

Cycling does not usually affect back pain recovery, but it conditions the body well. The indoor cross-country skiing machines appear to be good for backs as well. However, the stair-stepping machines cause a forward lean and often aggravate a bad back. And rowing machines should be treated with great respect!

The most important rule to remember is to stop doing any motion that causes lingering pain. However, pain that clears instantly upon stopping must be worked through.

Stretching

You should make stretching a part of your daily life because there are many benefits you will derive from it, including:
- Reduction of muscle tension
- Relaxation of the body
- Improvement in coordination by allowing easier movement
- Increased ranges of motion by elongating the muscles and ligaments

- Help in the prevention of muscle sprains/strains
- Strenuous activities will become easier
- Promotion of circulation
- Improvement in your balance

Be sure to follow these guidelines for stretching:

- Allow 10 to 20 minutes per day for stretching exercises.
- Don't bounce.
- Stretch slowly to prevent muscle straining.
- Breathe easily. Never hold your breath.
- Hold each stretch for 25 to 30 seconds.
- Exhale for the last five seconds of the stretch.
- Never stretch up to the point of pain.

• • •

Chapter Six:

Relaxation

"Turn off the stress, anger and fear . .
Discover the inner peace."

The ability to relax in our stress-laden world
is absolutely vital. Some people learn to relax
too well. They actually drop out of society completely. However, those with no relaxation skills
are just as unfortunate. Their internalized
stress, frustration and negative emotions
become a disease-promoting process. What one
needs to find, of course, is a happy middle-
ground where benefits can be derived from
proper relaxation techniques.

How To Start Relaxing

The first and most basic concept of relaxation is to create boredom in your mind. This is a state where you're neither excited, wishful, hopeful, nor fearful. Then you must learn how to transport that command of boredom from the subconscious mind to the automatic controls within your nervous system where it can be acted upon. It is vital to be in command of your nervous system. Consider that stress stimulates the fight-or-flight mechanisms which increase muscle tension, heartrate and restlessness. And, at the same time, stress can interfere with the digestive process and other normal bodily functions. (Remember the "Distress Cycle" shown in Diagram 2 in Chapter One?)

How many times have you tried to eat when rushed or stressed out, only to suffer later from acute indigestion? Need I say any more regarding the importance of mastering the ability to relax?

What Relaxation Does

When utilized correctly, the techniques of relaxation shorten the time the body needs to wind down after a stressful occurrence, be that a business meeting or a hard day at work. Hopefully, there is a quiet place where you can lie stretched out on your back in order to take advantage of correct relaxation techniques.

Set aside 15 to 20 minutes for "relaxation time" and try to take advantage of that time as soon as you get home from a stress-filled day. Once you are cognizant of correct relaxation techniques, you can relax any time, anywhere, at will! Stress will not be able to disarm you by piling up and causing pain.

For your convenience, I have outlined the following relaxation method and urge you to copy it for easy reference. If you use this method often enough, you will be able to commit it to memory and be well on your way toward learning a marvelous relaxation procedure.

1) First, get comfortable! Lie on your back with your arms at your sides. Once you're comfortable, say to yourself: "I am relaxed and safe." Believe what you are saying.

Repeat "I am relaxed and safe" slowly and rhythmically for five minutes the first day, 10 minutes the second day and 15 minutes the third day.

2) On day four, after the first five minutes, add this command: "My right arm weighs a ton." Repeat this in the same rhythmical monotone inner voice. Never speak aloud. Repeat this command for the last 10 minutes. What you are trying to do is achieve a true sense of having a heavy arm. If you are left-handed, substitute "left" for "right."

Within a few days, if you follow these steps, you will attain a relaxed and safe feeling in less than five minutes. You are aiming to create the feeling that your dominant arm could fall separately to the floor if it were not attached to your body.

When you reach this stage of progress, add this third command:

3) "My right (or left) arm is warm." Each session should last for 15 minutes, with the final command occupying the last 10. The first three commands are repeated in order and in the time interval it takes to actually experience the feeling commanded. This should take no more than five minutes per command after a few months of daily practice. At this stage you should be experiencing a very relaxed state and simultaneously be stopping the ill effects of your stress. Your back muscles should be unwinding, as should your stress-related attitudes and behavior patterns. At this point you should be a lot more fun to be around. (Your friends or mate will probably thank you.)

4) When your arm actually begins to feel warm, add this next command: "My circulation is calm and strong." As you repeat this command, visualize your blood calmly, but strongly, flowing from your heart through your body. You should experience a warm feeling all over.

5) When your body does indeed feel warm, add this command: "My forehead is colder." Repeat this command until your forehead feels colder than the rest of your body. You will be calm, relaxed, with your body feeling warm and your forehead cool, all achieved by your own command.

You *are* in total control.

If possible, try to practice the anti-stress method at approximately the same time each day. You are learning to relax, so don't try too hard. Let go and let it happen. Feel relaxed, safe and at peace before you do any of the other commands.

It takes months to progress from command one to five. When you finally achieve these commands, you will not only be more relaxed, you will feel quite pleased with your new skill. Being able to shift from out-of-control stress to healthy, automatic nervous controls is quite an achievement!

Your script for relaxation should look like the following. Remember, all these commands are repeated silently, with your calm, inner voice.

1) I AM RELAXED AND SAFE.

2) MY RIGHT/LEFT ARM WEIGHS A TON.

3) MY RIGHT/LEFT ARM IS WARM.

4) MY CIRCULATION IS CALM AND STRONG.

5) MY FOREHEAD IS COLDER THAN THE
REST OF MY BODY.

When you can achieve these sensations within a 15-minute period, and also shift from one sensation to another, then you can consider yourself an expert relaxer. What's more, once you have mastered it, you can utilize this method practically any time or any place.

If your daily routine permits, a good follow-up to a relaxation session is the stretching discussed in the previous chapter. If being over-weight is your problem, you may even discover your desire to eat is reduced to more normal levels by this discipline and new lifestyle addition. You'll be able to sit at a dining table in a relaxed mood. You won't need those rolls and butter to calm you down while you're waiting for the main course.

• • •

A large percentage of back pain sufferers are distressed. The combination of stress management as well as removing the mechanical dysfunctions is essential for long-lasting control of the pain.

Remember that good patients make good doctors. If you become an informed patient who is managing stress, it will be much easier to locate the right doctor who can help you become self-reliant. The best doctor-patient relationship for back sufferers can be likened to a coach-athlete relationship. Any doctor who does not help patients help themselves is creating a dependency that is doomed to failure.

Saying goodbye to back pain means changing your awareness of what is wrong with your back. Once you have the diagnosis, you will hopefully select the correct professional to provide rational, reasonable therapy. Moreover, you'll have a professional who can coach you through the necessary lifestyle changes that will allow you to attain your goal.

I look forward to hearing from you in the near future. Your success, problems and observations will be most valued in future editions of this book. You may write to me at the following address:

Dr. Leonard J. Faye
10780 Santa Monica Blvd.,
Suite 400
Los Angeles, CA 90025.

Before writing, give the whole relaxation method at least three months to work. And be sure to state the diagnosis of your particular back pain.

Keep in mind that success in alleviating your back pain is primarily up to you. You should now appreciate that many factors are involved in the deceptively simple complaint of back pain. If you underestimate the complexity of your problem you'll end up hopping from doctor to doctor. The surgeon may be waiting patiently at the end of the line, but with the right help, you can let him wait forever!

By now you not only know how you can relieve your own back pain, you also know why you or your doctor failed in previous attempts. If you're still not sure, go back and re-read what you don't understand. Because after mastering the techniques found within these pages, you too will say: *Good Bye Back Pain!*

•   •   •